Upper Urinary Tract Urothelial Carcinoma

Michael Grasso III • Demetrius H. Bagley
Editors

Upper Urinary Tract Urothelial Carcinoma

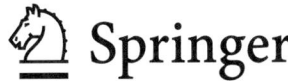 Springer

Editors
Michael Grasso III
Lenox Hill Hospital
Department of Urology
New York Medical College
Valhala, NY
USA

Demetrius H. Bagley
Department of Urology
Thomas Jefferson University
Philadelphia, PA
USA

ISBN 978-3-319-37142-9   ISBN 978-3-319-13869-5   (eBook)
DOI 10.1007/978-3-319-13869-5

Springer Cham Heidelberg New York Dordrecht London

Printed on acid-free paper

Springer International Publishing AG Switzerland is part of Springer Science+Business Media
(www.springer.com)

Preface

Recently, there have been changes in the diagnosis, treatment, and overall management of upper tract urothelial carcinoma. Although there have been suggestions that there is an increased frequency of these lesions, it is difficult to be certain because renal carcinoma and renal pelvic tumors are grouped together by coding. General success of various treatments in the lower urinary tract with preservation of the bladder leave the upper urinary tract naïve to intravesical therapies. Thus, it may remain as a reservoir of untreated urothelial tissue. The many studies of nephrectomy for renal cell carcinoma have demonstrated the value of preserving nephrons. This has been extended to increase the urgency of preservation with urothelial carcinoma as well.

The presentation of upper urinary tract urothelial carcinoma (UTUC) may be very nonspecific with hematuria as the most common finding. Radiographic studies may be indicative but are rarely definitive. Cytology and urinary markers similarly are often not diagnostic or specific. Endoscopic diagnosis is thus essential, most commonly requiring meticulous inspection of the upper tract urothelium with a steerable, flexible ureteropyeloscope and biopsy of any lesion detected.

As in the bladder, UTUC can present in various forms, some of which have a local indolent course (i.e., of lower grade) while others are aggressively malignant from the onset. Differentiating lesions based on endoscopic findings, urine cytology, and biopsies obtained with progressively small-diameter, mechanically refined ureteroscopes is essential in developing a treatment strategy. Genetic differentiation remains in its infancy. These same small-caliber ureteroscopes can then be employed to deliver a variety of energy sources to treat both ureteral and intrarenal lesions. Recurrence after endoscopic therapy parallels the lower urinary experience, underscoring the need for surveillance and the importance of developing adjuvant topical and systemic treatments.

While low-grade lesions can be treated endoscopically with organ preservation, high-grade and invasive lesions are most commonly treated with extirpative laparoscopic and surgical procedures. In these patients, there are significant risks of regional and widely metastatic disease, many of which might benefit from systemic chemotherapy before or after nephrectomy. Thus, it is the risk of transformation, or progression in grade, with a recurrence after endoscopic therapy of a low-grade lesion that is of paramount importance, framing an argument for lifelong surveillance protocols.

With diagnostic and treatment strategies evolving, based in part on new technologies and expanding experience, a comprehensive collaborative text focusing on upper tract urothelial carcinoma is timely. In this volume, authoritative specialists from various disciplines present a balanced scientific and practical approach to each subject.

New York, NY, USA   Michael Grasso III
Philadelphia, PA, USA   Demetrius H. Bagley

Contents

Contributors

Editors

Demetrius H. Bagley, MD Department of Urology, Thomas Jefferson University, Philadelphia, PA, USA

Michael Grasso III, MD Department of Urology, New York Medical College, Valhalla, New York, USA

Authors

Bobby S. Alexander, MD Department of Urology, Lenox Hill Hospital, New York, NY, USA

Christophe B. Anderson, MD Urology Service, Department of Surgery, Memorial Sloan Kettering Cancer Center, New York, NY, USA

Marluce Bibbo, MD, ScD Department of Pathology, Thomas Jefferson University, Philadelphia, PA, USA

Bruce M. Boman, MD, PhD Department of Medical Oncology, Thomas Jefferson University, Philadelphia, PA, USA

Mieke T.J. Bus, MD Department of Urology, Academic Medical Center, University of Amsterdam, Amsterdam, The Netherlands

Jonathan Cloutier, MD, FRCSC Department of Urology, Tenon University Hospital, Hôpitaux de Paris, Pierre et Marie Curie University, Paris, France

Michael J. Conlin, MD, MCR, FACS OHSU Center for Health and Healing, Oregon Health and Science University, Portland, OR, USA

Daniel Martin de Bruin, PhD Department of Urology, Academic Medical Center, University of Amsterdam, Amsterdam, The Netherlands

Department of Biomedical Engineering and Physics, Academic Medical Center, University of Amsterdam, Amsterdam, The Netherlands

Theo M. de Reijke, MD, PhD Department of Urology, Academic Medical Center, University of Amsterdam, Amsterdam, The Netherlands

Jean J.M.C.H. de la Rosette, MD, PhD Department of Urology, Academic Medical Center, University of Amsterdam, Amsterdam, The Netherlands

Brian Duty, MD OHSU Center for Health and Healing, Oregon Health and Science University, Portland, OR, USA

Andrew I. Fishman, MD Department of Urology, New York Medical College, Valhalla, NY, USA

Kelly Healy, MD Department of Urology, Thomas Jefferson University, Philadelphia, PA, USA

John Michael Henderson, BMBS, BMedSci(Hons), FRCS, FEBU Bristol Urological Institute, Southmead Hospital, Bristol, UK

Harry W. Herr, MD Urology Service, Department of Surgery, Memorial Sloan Kettering Cancer Center, New York, NY, USA

Jean Hoffman-Censits, MD Department of Medical Oncology, Kimmel Cancer Center, Thomas Jefferson University Hospital, Philadelphia, PA, USA

Scott G. Hubosky, MD Department of Urology, Thomas Jefferson University, Philadelphia, PA, USA

Gary Israel, MD Diagnostic Radiology, Yale New Haven Hospital, New Haven, CT, USA

Guido M. Kamphuis, MD Department of Urology, Academic Medical Center, University of Amsterdam, Amsterdam, The Netherlands

Francis X. Keeley Jr. , MD, FRCS (Urol) Bristol Urological Institute, Southmead Hospital, Bristol, UK

Costas D. Lallas, MD Department of Urology, Thomas Jefferson University, Philadelphia, PA, USA

Marc J. Mann, MD Department of Urology, Thomas Jefferson University, Philadelphia, PA, USA

John E. Musser, MD Department of Surgery, Memorial Sloan Kettering Cancer Center, New York, NY, USA

Lynn J. Paik, DO Department of Urology, Lenox Hill Hospital, New York, NY, USA

Shuyue Ren, MD, PhD Department of Pathology, Anatomy and Cell Biology, Thomas Jefferson University, Philadelphia, PA, USA

John P. Sfakianos, MD Department of Surgery, Memorial Sloan Kettering Cancer Center, New York, NY, USA

Sarah L. Steenbergen, MD Diagnostic Radiology, Yale New Haven Hospital, New Haven, CT, USA

Ryuta Tanimoto, MD Department of Urology, Thomas Jefferson University, Philadelphia, PA, USA

Edouard J. Trabulsi, MD, FACS Department of Urology, Kimmel Cancer Center, Sidney Kimmel Medical College, Thomas Jefferson University, Philadelphia, PA, USA

Oliver Traxer, MD, PhD Department of Urology, Tenon University Hospital, Hôpitaux de Paris, Pierre et Marie Curie University, Paris, France

Luca Villa, MD Department of Urology, Universita Vita-Salute San Raffaele, San Raffaele Hospital, Milan, Italy

Upper Tract Urothelial Carcinoma: Ureteroscopic Biopsy and Specimen Preparation

Demetrius H. Bagley, Ryuta Tanimoto, and Kelly A. Healy

Abbreviations

BTA	Bladder tumor antigen
CKD	Chronic kidney disease
CROES	Clinical research office of the endourological society
CSS	Cancer specific survival
F	French
FDP	Fibrin/fibrinogen degradation product
FISH	Fluorescence in situ hybridization
FU	Flexible ureteroscope
H & E	Hematoxylin and eosin
Ho	Holmium
MDCTU	Multidetector computed tomographic urography
NBI	Narrow band imaging
Nd	Neodymium
OS	Overall survival
PHH3	Phospho-histone H3
RNU	Radical nephroureterectomy
RPG	Retrograde ureteropyelogram
SPIES	Storz Professional Imaging Enhancement System
TUR	Transurethral resection
UTUC	Upper tract urothelial carcinoma
WL	White light
YAG	Yttrium aluminum garnet

1.1 Epidemiology

Upper tract urothelial carcinoma is relatively rare. Although urothelial carcinomas are the fourth most common tumor, most of these are located in the urinary lower urinary tract and upper tract urothelial carcinoma (UTUC) accounts for only 5 % of urothelial tumors and 8 % of renal tumors [1, 2]. In Western countries, the estimated annual incidence of UTUC is approximately 1–2 new cases per 100,000 inhabitants. The peak incidence occurs in people in their 70s and 80s and it is three times more prevalent in men than women. Concurrent bladder cancer is present in 8–13 % of cases. After treatment recurrent disease develops in the bladder in 15–50 % of UTUC tumor patients [3] (see Chap. 10). Tumors developed in the contralateral upper tract in 2–6 % of patients [4, 5].

There are several modifiable risk factors related to UTUC. Cigarette smoking is by far the most important of these, producing an incidence three times that seen in non-smokers [6]. Coffee consumption and analgesic abuse have been reported as risk factors [7, 8]. Environmental

D.H. Bagley, MD (✉) • R. Tanimoto, MD
K.A. Healy, MD
Department of Urology, Thomas Jefferson University, 1025 Walnut Street, Suite 1112 College Building, Philadelphia, PA 19107, USA
e-mail: Demetrius.bagley@jefferson.edu

© Springer International Publishing Switzerland 2015
M. Grasso III, D.H. Bagley (eds.), *Upper Urinary Tract Urothelial Carcinoma*,
DOI 10.1007/978-3-319-13869-5_1

factors exhibited in employment exposures can be extremely important and risky. Exposure for those employed in the chemical, petroleum, or plastic industries has been seen to increase the relative risk to four. Exposure to coal or coke increases the risk by fourfold. Those exposed to asphalt or tar have a relative risk of 5.5. Aniline dyes, beta-naphthyamine and benzidine have also been associated as causative.

Ingestion of aristolochic acid as a Chinese medicinal herb or as a component of other medical compounds has been related to higher risk of UTUC and has even been responsible for a shift in the sex preponderance in populations where the medicines are popular. With all environmentally related neoplasms there may be a multi-year lag after exposure, up to 15 years or more.

There are also familial or hereditary cases of UTUC. The most common of these is non-polyposis colorectal carcinoma (HNPCC). This is described later in Chap. 10.

1.2 Symptoms

There are really very few symptoms related to the presence of upper tract urothelial carcinoma. By far, the most common presentation is observation of gross or microscopic hematuria (73–78 %). Flank pain may occur in up to 18–32 % of cases. It is generally dull or achy and is thought to be secondary to a gradual onset of obstruction and hydronephrosis. Less commonly pain may be acute and similar to renal colic. This is typically associated with the passage of clots that obstruct the collecting system [5, 9]. About 15 % of patients are totally asymptomatic at presentation and are diagnosed when an incidental lesion is found on radiologic evaluation. Patients also may have only late symptoms with advanced disease, such as flank or abdominal mass, weight loss, anorexia, and bone pain. There is no difference in prognosis between patients who have preoperative symptoms and those who remain symptom free. Systemic symptoms including anorexia, weight loss, malaise, fatigue, fever, night sweats, or cough associated with UTUC are more commonly associated with advanced disease and should raise concern for a thorough metastatic evaluation and consideration of perioperative chemotherapy regimens [10].

1.3 Options in Treatment

The majority of UTUC are invasive at the time of diagnosis compared to only 15 % of bladder tumors [9, 11, 12]. Overall 5-year cancer specific survival (CSS) is approximately 75 % but is highly stage dependent. The 5-year CSS exceeds 90 % for pTa and T1 disease, it declines to 74.7 %, 54 %, and 12.2 % for pT2, pT3, and pT4 disease, respectively [13]. These differences in survival are seen with radical surgical nephroureterectomy, laparoscopic resection or endoscopic treatment. While radical nephroureterectomy with bladder cuff incision has been the gold standard for UTUC, the options are changing. Radical nephroureterectomy can be performed using an open, laparoscopic or robotic assisted approach.

However, about half of patients with UTUC have pre-existing renal insufficiency with GFR less than 60 mL/min/1.73 m [14]. With advances in ureteroscopes as well as ablative devices, ureteroscopic resection has emerged as an attractive alternative nephron-sparing option in carefully selected patients with acceptable long-term outcomes [15–17]. Though initially reserved for patients with absolute indications for nephron preservation [18–21], ureteroscopic management is now electively done in those with a normal contralateral kidney [22, 23] with renal maintenance in approximately 70–80 % of cases [20, 24]. Recently, the risks of chronic kidney disease (CKD) have become increasingly recognized and CKD is associated with a wide range of causes of increased mortality, particularly cardiovascular [25–27]. As such, emphasis has been placed on nephron preservation, specifically partial nephrectomy for renal cell carcinoma [28–30]. These same arguments can be extrapolated to UTUC. The concept of renal preservation is also appealing due to the risk of panurothelial recurrences. The appropriate selection of patients for conservative management is imperative. Currently, accurate staging remains a challenge and grade serves as a surrogate for stage. Thus, obtaining an accurate tissue diagnosis is a critical step in the decision making process for UTUC patients.

1.4 Imaging Studies

Multidetector computed tomographic urography (MDTCU) is presently the imaging standard for evaluation of the upper urinary tract [31–35]. It has been seen to be extremely accurate to identify lesions. For polypoid tumors between five and 10 mm, it has a sensitivity of 96 % and specificity of 99 %. Sensitivity decreases to 89 % for lesions less than 5 mm and 40 % for polyploid lesions less than 3 mm but flat lesions are considerably more difficult to diagnose until they become massive. However, CT has the advantage of providing staging information.

Magnetic resonance urography (MRU) can be used in patients who cannot have a CT scan because of contrast allergy or azotemia [37]. It does appear to be less sensitive with the detection rate of only 75 % for tumors <2 cm [38]. It also is generally considered to be contraindicated in patients with severe renal impairment (creatinine clearance <30 mL/min) because of the risk of the very rare nephrogenic systemic fibrosis [39]. Other options in imaging include excretory urography or retrograde ureteropyelography, possibly combined with noncontrast CT scan or renal ultrasound to search for both intraluminal filling defects and renal masses.

Several reports have noted that hydronephrosis is an ominous sign predicting higher grade and stage tumors [36, 40, 41].

Imaging studies alone are not adequate to diagnose UTUC definitively. Numerous benign lesions may cause filling defects including polyp, blood clot, fungus ball, inflammatory lesion, or noncalcified radiolucent lesion such as a matrix calculus. Ureteral endoscopy is necessary in these patients to define the subject lesion. Endoscopic visualization alone cannot provide the exact diagnosis. Endoscopic appearance was accurate in only 70 % of patients to determine the malignancy or grade of an upper tract tumor in one series [42]. In another, patients with only a visual endoscopic diagnosis developed grade 3 UTUC during follow up in 21 % [43] indicating the inadequacy of inspection alone.

The decision for treatment can be based to some extent on the tumor grade which reflects the tumor stage. Low-grade, low volume tumors have responded well to endoscopic treatment. With overall survival and cancer specific survival equivalent to that achieved with radical nephroureterectomy in low grade and stage disease. Those with high-grade disease do poorly with either approach [15, 18]. Ureteroscopy with biopsy and possibly simultaneous resection has been the most accurate technique so far for grading and also possibly staging, as well as treating upper tract lesions [44–46].

Herein, we describe our techniques for the ureteroscopic biopsy and specimen handling of upper urinary tract tumors. In doing so, patients may be appropriately selected for a nephronsparing ureteroscopic laser ablation versus extirpative surgery with RNU and bladder cuff excision for the management of UTUC.

1.5 Urine Based Markers in Diagnosis of UTUC

The ideal diagnostic study for UTUC would be from voided urine collected noninvasively which could demonstrate both high sensitivity and specificity. Unfortunately, no currently available marker fulfills these criteria. Numerous immunologic studies and assays for urinary proteins have failed to achieve better accuracy than cytology alone. Several improved sensitivity and/or specificity when added to cytology but not to the point that would allow treatment without endoscopic biopsy.

Cytology of voided urine has been shown to have a sensitivity of only 30 % for the detection of bladder cancer. The sensitivity varies by grade: Grade one was 12 %, grade two 26 % and grade three 64 % [47]. Cytology is even less sensitive to detect UTUC [48]. Other techniques have been employed in an attempt to enhance the yield for cytology for upper tract tumors. Bibbo et al. used urine obtained from the upper tract with ureteral catheterization and barbotage or brushing and found an improvement of the sensitivity of cytology for UTUC [49]. Thus, they demonstrated the value of direct sampling of tumors in the upper tract. Those particular techniques have been replaced with endoscopic biopsy.

Several urine based markers have been employed for the diagnosis and follow-up of urothelial carcinoma. In general, these have shown superior sensitivities but higher false-positive rates compared to cytology [47, 50, 51]. At least 18 urine-based tests for urothelial carcinoma of bladder have become available. (BTAstat, BTAtrak, NMP22, FDP, ImmunoCyt, Cytometry, Quanticyt, Hb-dipstick, LewisX, FISH, Telomerase, Microsatellite, CYFRA21-1, UBC, Cytokeratin20, BTA, TPS, Cytology). Based on the specificity and sensitivity of urine markers solely for UCC surveillance, Microsatellite analysis, ImmunoCyt, NMP22, CYFRA21-1, LewisX and FISH are the most promising markers for surveillance of UCC [50]. Among UTUC patients, select studies have assessed the utility of alternative markers including Immunocyt™, NMP22, bladder tumor antigen (BTA), fibrin/fibrinogen degradation product (FDP), and fluorescence in situ hybridization (FISH).

As an immunocytochemical diagnostic tool, Immunocyt™ traces three monoclonal antibodies (19A211, M344, and LDQ10) which are directed against three antigens (two mucins and a carcinoembryonic antigen) expressed on urothelial carcinoma [52]. In carcinoma of the bladder, Immunocyt™ had an overall sensitivity and specificity for voided urine of 86.1 % and 80 %, respectively. It maintained a higher sensitivity (84–96 %) than cytologic analysis (4–56 %) for grades 1 and 2 tumors [52, 53]. Lodde et al. studied the use of Immunocyt™ in 37 patients with suspected UTUC [54]. They found a higher overall sensitivity for detecting UTUC compared to cytology in voided and ureteral urine. Comparison of Immunocyt™ and voided urine cytology showed that it was more sensitive at detecting grade 1 (33 % vs. 0 %) and 2 (100 % vs. 17 %). In grade 3, this was reversed and Immunocyt™ was less than cytology (71 % vs. 100 %).

Combination of cytology and Immunocyt™ yielded very high results with 100 % sensitivity and specificity. The authors concluded that Immunocyt™ complements cytology in detecting UTUC, mainly because of its high sensitivity for low grade tumors.

NMP22 is a nuclear protein that is responsible for the chromatid regulation and cell separation during replication. This is a quantitative ELISA assay that requires urine stabilization. The sensitivity of the NMP22 test in separated and voided urine was 73.2 and 70.5 %, respectively, compared to 64.7 and 58.8 % of urine cytology. The specificity of the NMP22 test in separated and voided urine was 88 and 92 %, respectively, compared to 96 and 96 % of urine cytology. There is a high agreement of the NMP22 test in voided and separated urine, indicating that the voided urine is adequate for diagnosis [55].

The BTA test is a qualitative latex agglutination assay which detects the presence of basement membrane complexes exfoliated in the urine in patients with urothelial carcinoma [56–58]. Although several studies have shown that the BTA test is superior in sensitivity to urinary cytology for primary and recurrent bladder cancer, (ranging from 50 to 82 % [59, 60]), the BTA test was poor at identifying upper tract tumors. Zimmerman et al. using ureteroscopically sampled urine specimens found 60 % sensitivity and 40 % specificity of this test [56]. The authors then concluded that the BTA test did not have clinical value for diagnosing UTUC.

FDP detects urinary fibrin/fibrinogen degradation products in a lateral flow immunoassay using monoclonal antibodies. It was described to be sensitive in patients with bladder cancer [61–63]. FDP had a higher overall sensitivity (81 %) compared to either BTA (28 %) or urinary cytology (35 %) [63]. A preliminary prospective study found that FDP showed promise for both voided urine and ureteral washing in patients with upper tract urothelial carcinoma with an high sensitivity of 100 % (BTA 50 %, cytology 29 %) and accuracy of 83 % (BTA 62 %, cytology 59 %) but with a decreased specificity of 67 % (BTA 73 %, cytology 86 %) [61].

FISH assay uses fluorescent probes that detect four chromosomal anomalies typical in bladder cancer. These are chromosomes 3, 7, 17, and the 9p21 band [64, 65]. In studies of bladder cancer, FISH demonstrated higher sensitivity than cytology, but has not eliminated the need for direct cytoscopic evaluation to diagnose the bladder cancer [66–68]. Several studies have examined voided urine FISH to detect UTUC, but the sensitivity has varied widely from 35 to 87.5 % [69–72].

Three smaller studies showed a higher sensitivity but the majority of patients were treated with nephroureterectomy [69, 70]. Lodde et al. in his study of Immunocyt™ had 37 patients who were either symptomatic or had radiographic evidence of UTUC and found the sensitivity of 75 % [54]. However, 13 of the 16 patients confirmed to have UUTUC had extirpative surgery while only 3 were managed endoscopically. Akkad et al. found 87.5 % sensitivity in 16 patients with suspected UTUC [69]. Marin-Aguilera et al. found 76.7 % sensitivity of FISH but only 36 % for cytology [70]. Again, the majority of patients (21/30) were treated with radical nephroureterectomy. This high rate of surgical treatment raises the question of whether the patients demonstrating positive markers or even cytology may represent those with high volume and higher grade disease.

Other larger series have questioned the value of voided FISH in diagnosing UTUC. Mian et al. evaluated the reliability of FISH for UTUC in 55 consecutive patients. The overall sensitivity of the cytology was 20.8 % and of FISH 100 %. The specificity was 97.4 % for cytology and 89.5 % for FISH [73]. Chen and Grasso evaluated 94 FISH specimens from voided urine or selective samples obtained endoscopically in patients with upper tract tumors [71]. Voided specimens demonstrated a poor sensitivity of 35 % but it improved for bladder washings and selective upper tract washings to 67 % and 65 %, respectively. It appears that invasive sampling may increase the diagnostic yield, but still FISH alone cannot function as a reliable noninvasive test for the detection of UTUC. In 8 studies of FISH and urine cytology for the detection of UTUC, the overall median sensitivity of the cytology was 31.0 % and of FISH 85.7 %, while the median specificity was 97.4 % for cytology and 93.9 % for FISH [69–77]. When used for detection of UTUC after cystectomy, both FISH and urinary cytology demonstrate high rates of false positivity. They may be helpful for their negative predictive ability in patients with a urinary diversion [78]. These combined results demonstrate that voided FISH did not provide adequate sensitivity and specificity to eliminate direct ureteroscopic evaluation.

No currently available urine-based markers summarized are adequate to provide a definite diagnosis for initial evaluation or surveillance of UTUC. Direct endoscopic inspection and sampling remains the best diagnostic study and also provides an opportunity to treat selected low volume, low grade tumors.

1.6 Tissue-Based Markers for UTUC

Recently, biomarkers have been studied to search for biologically aggressive tumors and to define the prognosis of patients with UTUC. Various studies have evaluated tissue-based markers related to cellular processes such as cell adhesion (E-cadherin, β-catenin, Parvin-β, CD24), angiogenesis (HIF-1α, Metalloproteinases), cell proliferation (Ki-67 EGFR, Uroplakin3, Snail) and apoptosis (p53, Bcl-2, Survivin) [79]. Many of these studies have been limited by the rarity of UTUC and with subsequent small sample size. Two prospective studies looked at the usefulness of tissues-based biomarkers for prognosis of UTUC. Bagrodia et al. used a panel of tissue biomarkers for cell cycle regulators (p53, p21, p27, cyclin E) and a proliferative marker (Ki-67) in 73 patients with UTUC treated by radical nephroureterectomy. These were grouped into favorable and unfavorable by the number of altered biomarkers: 0–2-favorable; >2 unfavorable. The unfavorable marker profile was associated with advanced pathologic T stage, non-organ confined disease, LVI and tumor necrosis. Among patients with an unfavorable profile, 70.9 % had T3/T4 tumors while only 23.8 % of the favorable cohort (p<0.001) had the higher stage. Similarly, there was a higher rate of LN involvement in the unfavorable score group (25.8 % vs 9.5 %, p=0.06). Cancer-specific survival was significantly longer for patients with a favorable biomarker score (41.1 months vs 28.9 months; p=0.04). These authors suggested that biomarker analysis of specimens might commit selective use of neoadjuvant chemotherapy and more extended lymphadenectomy at the time of RNU [80]. Krabbe et al. [81] studied Ki-67 over expression in 101 consecutive patients with high grade UTUC after RNU. Ki-67 over expression was associated with worse pathological features (T stage, nonorgan confined disease, LVI and sessile architecture). Those patients with over expression had significantly worse recurrence-free survival (43.2 vs 69.0 months, p=0.006) and cancer specific survival (48.9 vs 68.9 months, p=0.031) than patients with normal Ki-67. Even after adjustment for the effects of organ vs nonorgan confined disease, Ki-67 over expression was an independent predictor of recurrence-free survival in the total group (HR 4.3, p=0.05) and in patients with nonmetastatic disease (HR 8.5, p=0.038) [80]. These markers have not been defined from endoscopic biopsy but if the same findings develop, there is the potential for treatment plans to include neoadjuvant systemic chemotherapy and also to eliminate some treatment for patients who have limited benefits.

1.7 Endoscopic and Biopsy Techniques

Endoscopic evaluation of the entire urinary tract is essential in a patient being evaluated for first upper tract carcinoma or in surveillance after previous treatment. Cystoscopy is first performed to visualize the entire urethra, prostate, and bladder. Cystoscopy is important since bladder tumors may present in the of newly diagnosed patients and may occur in 20–50 % after endoscopic treatment [82]. A urine sample from the bladder is obtained for cytology. When a rigid cystoscope is used, usually both a 30° and 70° telescope is

necessary to view the entire mucosa. A flexible cystoscope can also be used but it makes the retrograde ureteropyelogram more difficult. A retrograde should be performed on the affected and the contralateral side. Bilateral tumors for metachronous contralateral lesions may occur in 5–10 % of patients [82]. We prefer to use dilute (30 %) iodinated contrast (Fig. 1.1) with an appropriately sized cone tip catheter, usually 8 French. This type of catheter provides an excellent seal at the ureteral orifice preventing leakage of contrast into the bladder and allowing some distension of the collecting system. If there is some dilation of the orifice, then it may be necessary to use a 10 F cone tip catheter. A non-occluding catheter, such as an open-end or whistle-tip may not adequately distend the upper tract and may traumatize the urothelium. Great care must be taken to avoid over distension of the collecting system with the risk of extravastion. Over distension, as with excessively dense contrast material, may also obscure filling defects.

Unless there is a finding on the contralateral ureteropyelogram, endoscopy is limited to the suspicious affected side. One of two "no touch techniques" is employed. This describes endoscopic inspection of the entire urothelium prior to any instrumentation. No guidewire which can traumatize the urothelium and the first and

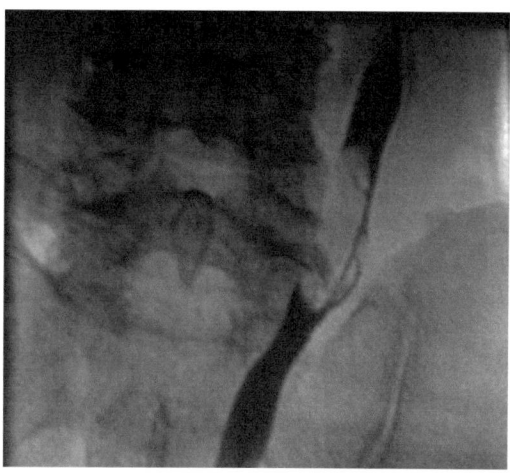

Fig. 1.1 A retrograde with 30 % iodinated contrast mildly dilates and clearly outlines the ureter and the filling defect of the 3 cm neoplasm

the earliest "no touch technique," uses a small caliber rigid ureteroscope passed through the bladder and into the ureteral orifice under direct vision [83, 84]. The endoscope is advanced as far proximally as possible without excessive torque or angulation. Often in a female, the ureteroscope can be passed to the renal pelvis without difficulty, and the endoscope typically cannot be passed beyond the level of the mid-ureter at the iliac vessels in most patients. This initial passage of the radially dilating semi-rigid ureteroscope to inspect the distal and mid ureter mildly dilates the ureteral orifice and distal ureter and facilitates insertion of the flexible ureteroscope (FU). A guidewire is then passed through the rigid ureteroscope and left in place only to the most proximal level of the ureter inspected. The position of the wire is confirmed, both endoscopically and fluoroscopically. Strict attention should be taken to prevent inadvertent proximal migration of the wire. Dilation of the ureter should also be avoided to minimize trauma to the ureter from or the dilation itself. It is rarely necessary to dilate. Hudson et al. described that the ideal flexible ureteroscope outer diameter is 7.5 French (F) to minimize the need for ureteric dilation since <1 % of cases failed to pass using this size scope [85]. Flexible ureteroscopes from most manufacturers have increased in size to 8.3–8.5 F. Some digital ureteroscopes are even larger and may require dilation.

In the second "no touch technique", the flexible ureteroscope is used alone without any initial rigid endoscopy. With the appropriate size ureter and flexible ureteroscope, it can be inserted directly into the ureteral orifice in a wireless, sheathless approach [86]. The flexible ureteroscope is passed through the urethra and bladder and then directly into the ureteral orifice. It is passed throughout the ureter to inspect the entire mucosa and then into the intrarenal collecting system.

As with the rigid technique, vision must be maintained through the passage of the flexible ureteroscope. Any small ureteral tumors are biopsied and treated as they are encountered using the techniques described below (Fig. 1.2). Such small lesions at 1–3 mm may be avulsed

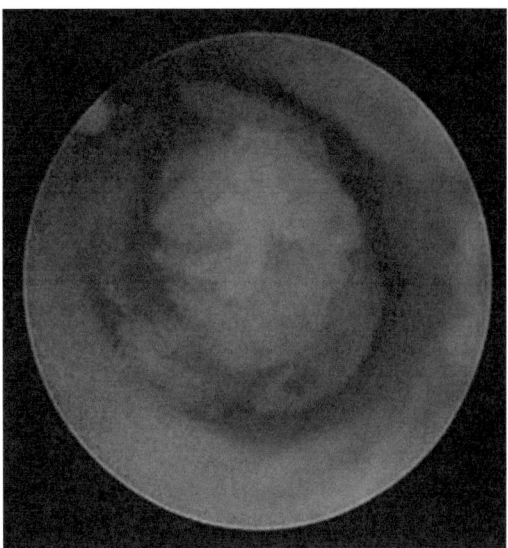

Fig. 1.2 Ureteral tumors visualized during initial ureteroscopy are sampled and treated to avoid damage and loss from instrumentation

with scope advancement and be lost or possibly induce bleeding. Therefore, they are treated as they are encountered. If, in comparison, a large lesion is found, it may be helpful to advance the ureteroscope beyond the lesion into the more proximal ureteral segment to identify other tumors.

With larger tumors such as those that fill the lumen and may extend 1–2 cm beyond the base (e.g. Fig. 1.1), it may be difficult to identify the ureteral lumen itself to get past the tumor. It may be useful to follow the contour of the ureteral wall or, in select cases, pass a hydromer coated guidewire beyond the tumor to gain proximal access. Although a "no touch technique" is preferred, a guidewire is used whenever it is needed to ensure access.

Next, the ureteroscope is advanced into the renal pelvis. An aspirate of urine is obtained and sent for cytology. This is completed by connecting a large (50–60 mL) Luer lock syringe directly to the irrigation port (Fig. 1.3). Avoid touching the pelvis and certainly avoid aspirating against the mucosa to avoid traumatic bleeding. The collecting system is then inspected systematically. First the entire pelvis is seen and then the intrarenal collecting system. Since severe deflection may be required to reach lower pole calices thus

Fig. 1.3 Renal pelvic urine and irrigant is aspirated from the pelvis through the channel of the ureteroscope

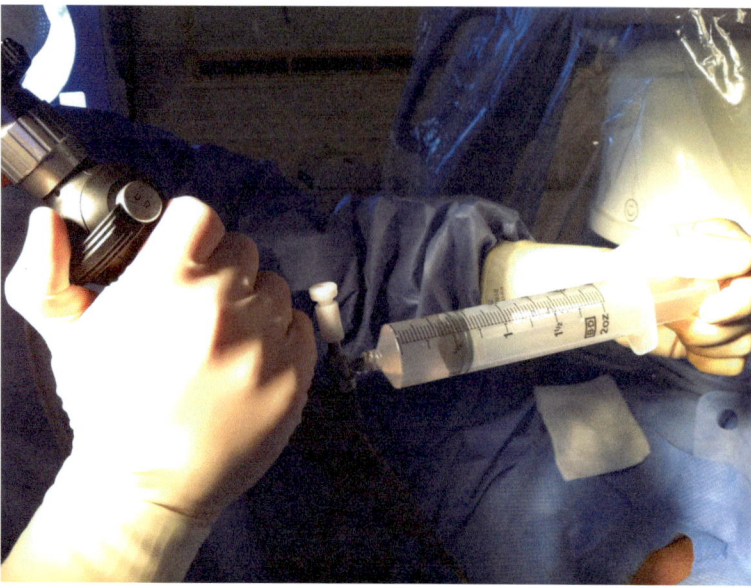

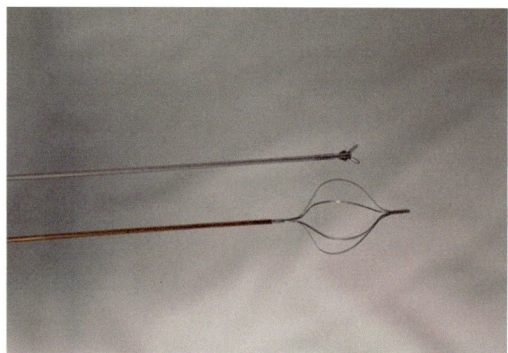

Fig. 1.4 A 1 mm biopsy forceps and a flat wire basket are commonly used for ureteroscopic biopsy [87]

inducing bleeding, inspection should proceed from the renal pelvis to the upper, mid and finally the lower calices.

Any tumors seen within the renal collecting system are biopsied and possibly treated at the end of the inspection. Various devices have been introduced to biopsy upper tract tumors, including baskets, forceps, brushes, snares and graspers. The most successful and most commonly used devices are the 3 French cup biopsy forceps and the stainless steel flat wire basket [87] (Fig. 1.4). The cup forceps are available in several designs of 1 mm diameter. These are well suited for sampling smaller papillary lesions, ses-

sile or flat lesions. If the sample is entirely contained within the cup, the device can be withdrawn through the working channel. The device is then replaced through the ureteroscope and multiple samples are taken in a similar fashion to ensure a sufficient specimen for cytologic evaluation. If the tissue fragment extends beyond the cup, the entire unit consisting of FU, forceps, and biopsy specimen should be removed from the collecting system to preserve the largest specimen possible. The endoscope is then replaced and additional biopsies are obtained.

Depending on the ureteroscope employed and cup forceps, the device may limit the deflection to only 90–100° [82]. This may prevent positioning to biopsy lower pole lesions.

The stainless steel flat wire basket is quite effective for more sizable, papillary, and friable tumors [83, 87]. The tumor is visualized and the basket extended and applied to the tumor itself. It is manipulated to bury the wires into the tumor and the basket is then closed snugly but not completely, which would cut the sample from the basket. It is used to avulse a piece of tissue. In this way, a large sample measuring up to several millimeters may be retrieved. These larger samples should not be withdrawn through the working channel since most of the tissue would be sheared off and lost. Instead, the entire unit consisting of FU, basket, and biopsy should always be withdrawn to maintain the largest tissue specimen possible (Fig. 1.5). The FU is reinserted and multiple biopsies are taken. With this flat wire technique, large tumors up to several cm in diameter can be mechanically debulked quite effectively. Kleinmann et al. compared the flat wire basket and cup biopsy forceps for the success rate of diagnosis and grade determination of UTUC. Diagnosis was successful in 63 and 94 % (P < 0.0001) and specific grade was determined in 80 and 93 % (P = 0.033) in the forceps and basket groups, respectively. On subgroup analysis of tumors larger than 10 mm in diameter, the flat wire basket was still shown to be superior in achieving pathologic diagnosis (P = 0.037) [87].

Other devices are relatively ineffective and are rarely used in our practice. The nitinol round wire baskets, described as atraumatic, do not have enough grasping edge to capture tumor well. The brush is also very poor in retrieving tissue. When it is viewed directly endoscopically, the brush can be seen moving the tissue but not actually sampling it. It should be recalled, however, that cystoscopic placement of the brush to a filling defect improved sampling and diagnostic capability over voided urine alone [49]. Wire pronged graspers cause less loss of deflection with the flexible ureteroscope and may be used to sample tumors in the lower pole. However, the device cannot adequately sample or retrieve the tissue. More often, the prongs will tear off bits of the tissue which may be able to be retrieved by aspirating through the channel of the endoscope.

Recently, a cup forceps with a larger 2 mm cup has been introduced. Because of the size of the cup, the device must be back-loaded through the working channel of the FU. Subsequently, the flexible ureteroscope with the back-loaded forceps must be placed through a ureteral access sheath. If this technique is employed, we strongly recommend inspecting the ureter first with a "no touch technique" to evaluate for ureteral lesions prior to placing the access sheath. Next, it will be noted that the large cup forceps obscure the visual field. This device appears to have a more flexible shaft which allows better deflection. Although the sample achieved with the 2 mm forceps is greater than with the 1 mm, it is much smaller than that which can be retrieved with a flat wire basket.

1.8 Handling of Specimen

The tissue sample obtained with any of these techniques is transferred directly from the cup forceps or basket into a specimen container with normal saline (Fig. 1.5). It should not be placed first into a container in the operative field and then changed to the final specimen container. By minimizing the number of transfers, the chance of loss of specimen is minimized. If the delivery of the specimen to the Cytopathology laboratory is delayed (such as at night), the specimen is placed in a container with Saccomanno fixative. Preferably, fresh specimens are hand delivered to the laboratory where they are evaluated using the Cytospin smear technique. Importantly, all samples are processed as cytology specimens to avoid tissue loss during preparation [88]. Multiple samples are taken with either device to obtain sufficient tissue for pathologic analysis. In addition to the biopsy samples themselves, post-biopsy and post-laser aspirates are obtained for cytology (Also see Chap. 4).

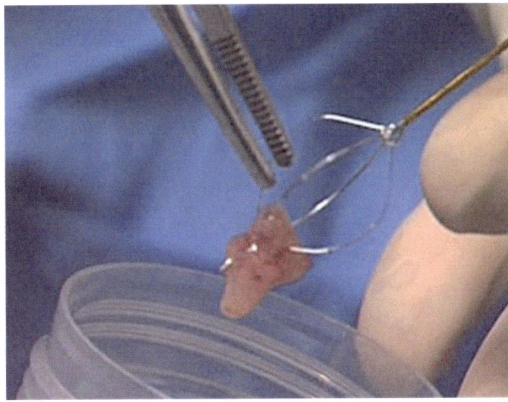

Fig. 1.5 The several mm tumor sample taken with the basket is transferred directly to the specimen cup containing saline. The sample can be lifted from the wires with forceps

1.9 Endoscopic Treatment

After biopsying the tumor adequately, it can be treated. It also should be noted that additional biopsy samples can be obtained, particularly if new or uninspected portions of the tumor are revealed during treatment. There are options among devices for endoscopic treatment. There are 2 and 3 F monopolar electrodes available which can be passed through the working channel of the flexible ureteroscope and powered by standard electrosurgical units available in almost any hospital. It may require special connecting cords which are generally available.

Lasers have assumed the dominant role in the endoscopic treatment of UTUC. The holmium (Ho) and neodymium (Nd):yttrium aluminum garnet (YAG) lasers have the largest role for treatment [82]. Some diode lasers have also been used. The Ho:YAG laser is a pulsed instrument with a wavelength of 2,100 nm. The energy from the Ho:YAG laser penetrates tissue only 0.5 mm so that its tissue effect is both superficial and visible endoscopically. It also must be positioned very close to the target tissue. This laser is primarily ablative but can also be used to coagulate tumors by defocusing the laser beam on the tissue by withdrawing it slightly from the target. Specific Ho:YAG lasers are available with a variable pulse duration. It is usually 350 μs but in those specific lasers can be increased to 700 μs. Its effect as seen as increasing coagulation. It also decreases the movement of stone during treatment.

The Nd:YAG laser has a continuous wave and a wavelength of 1,064 nm. Its penetration is deeper to approximately 5–10 mm. It is difficult to determine the depth of penetration so that it is best to follow its treatment in coagulation of tissue endoscopically. Both electrocautery and the Nd:YAG laser only coagulate tissue. The electrosurgical device must be in contact with the tissue while the Nd:YAG does not require contact, but in fact, can be a few mm from the tissue to be treated. Both should be used very carefully if at all in the ureter because of the risk of stricture formation. They should also be used very selectively within the kidney because of the risk of infundibular stenosis. Both are effective at coagulating bleeding sites. The Nd:YAG laser and less conveniently the electrocautery can be used in combination with the Ho:YAG laser. The tissue is first coagulated and then ablated with the Holmium.

The endoscopic treatment of tumor is discussed in greater depth in Chap. 5.

As noted above, all of the specimens which are at best small, are handled with cytopathologic techniques (Table 1.1). The specimens are delivered fresh in saline to the Cytopathology laboratory. The majority of the samples are prepared with the cytospin technique. If there is any macroscopically visible tissue in the sample, a cell block is also prepared. The latter can often demonstrate both of the architecture neoplasm and the individual cells to allow grading of urothelial carcinoma.

1.10 Cytospin Technique

The fresh specimen is prepared with Saccomanno fixative. If the specimen is grossly hematuric, a Cytorich red solution is added to lyse the red blood cells. The specimen is then centrifuged for 10 min at 1,200 RPM. Most of the supernatant is then discarded but 3–5 mL is placed into a special funnel apparatus, which contains a specimen slide, and again centrifuged for 10 min at 1,300 RPM. The cells are then adherent to the slide which is removed and air dried for 10 min. It is then placed in 95 % alcohol to remove the carbowax contained in the Saccomanno fixative and is subsequently inserted into the machine for Papanicolaou staining. The final step is to place the slide in Xylene bath for 2 min for clearing of the alcohol and then coverslipped.

Table 1.1 Samples Obtained During Endoscopic Biopsy

1. Bladder urine
2. Saline wash and aspirate from site of lesion
3. Biopsy of the lesion (in saline)
4. Post biopsy aspirate
5. Post laser aspirate

1.11   Cell Block Preparation

A cell block should be prepared whenever there is any macroscopically visible tissue in the sample. This is done with the pellet obtained following the first centrifugation. The pellet is transferred to a fenestrated bag and wet with formalin. The bag is wrapped and placed in a cassette, which is immersed in formalin solution. The specimen is processed in several solutions, including two fixations in formalin, dehydration from 70 % alcohol through three absolute alcohol solutions, and clearing of alcohol in Xylene solution. It is then extracted from the bag and embedded in wax, sliced, and adhered to a glass slide. Lastly, the slides are stained with hematoxylin and eosin (H & E) and prepared as a histologic specimen. Architectural and cellular details of the lesion can often be demonstrated using the cell block preparation just as a histologic specimen.

Prior to using these techniques with a systematic approach, even the larger endoscopic biopsies tended to get lost during preparation. By handling all specimens in the Cytopathology laboratory, our diagnostic yield increased from 40 % to approximately 90 %.

1.12   Other Staining Techniques

Alternative fixatives and preservatives solution as well as stains are being evaluated in an attempt to improve the diagnostic yield in ureteroscopic biopsies. Bultitude et al. assessed whether Bouin's fixative could improve the interpretation of ureteroscopic biopsies [89]. Bouin's is a non-coagulate picrate solution which is routinely utilized to fix testicular biopsies because it preserves the nuclear detail. In this series, 28 pathological areas were studied in 18 patients. There were two groups of patients: Bouin's group (7 patients, 10 pathological areas) versus 10 % Formalin group (11 patients, 18 pathological areas). The specimens were reviewed by two pathologists in a blinded fashion using an objective scoring system to evaluate five domains: specimen quality/size, specimen processing, architecture, cytoplasmic detail, and nuclear detail. No equivocal results were seen in the Bouin's group but there were two equivocal biopsies in the formalin group. Nuclear detail was better preserved in the samples fixed in Bouin's solution ($p < 0.001$).

The authors did note that Bouin's solution is useful as either a fixative or staining solution, but it is not suitable as a preservative because of tissue shrinkage induced by the picric acid, tissues cannot be stored in Bouin's solution for more than 48 h [89]. Also since the tissue is stained yellow, the solution makes specimen identification easier at the time of sampling and while embedding. The stain is removed with multiple ethanol washes. The authors concluded that Bouin's fixative improved the assessment of ureteroscopic biopsies particularly with better preservation of nuclear details.

Special stains are also being studied to improve the pathologic analysis of ureteroscopic biopsies. Grading of UTUC has been challenging for interobserver agreement. Both mitotic figure counting and nuclear features are important in tumor grading but several factors such as apoptosis and artifact may interfere. Solomides et al. studied the use of a mitotic specific marker phospho-histone H3 (PHH3) as an adjunct to H & E stain for grading UTUC in cell blocks [90]. Formalin fixed paraffin embedded cell blocks from 61 upper tract urothelial carcinomas were stained with H & E followed by PHH3-antibody. Three pathologists graded tumors in a blinded fashion, first on H & E and then on H & E plus PHH3 stained slides. Gradings were compared between pathologists for each group. By adding the PHH3 stain to the H & E stain, the interobserver agreement in grading among the three pathologists improved dramatically and was statistically significant (average pairwise agreement $= 80$ %, overall kappa $= 0.69$). Therefore, PHH3 immunostain may improve grading of UTUC in small cell block samples.

1.13   Assisted Imaging Techniques

The visual diagnosis and sampling of UTUC remains imperfect. White light (WL) imaging is limited as the only modality in detecting the presence and extent of urothelial lesions, both in the bladder and in the upper urinary tract. Other optical diagnostics have been introduced in an attempt to extend these limitations [91]. Narrow band imaging (NBI) has been employed to enhance the visualization of more vascular structures. Similarly, the SPIES (Storz Professional Imaging Enhancement System) is another imaging enhancement modality being studied to improve the visualization of urothelial carcinoma. These techniques are discussed in greater detail in Chaps. 12 and 13.

The accuracy of ureteroscopic biopsies in relation to the final findings on pathology, particularly the tumor grade has been concerning. Several studies have demonstrated a biopsy concordance of up to 80–90 % between the endoscopic and final pathologic specimens [43, 44]. It appears that the accuracy can be enhanced by multiple samples dispersed throughout the tumor and associated cytology specimen. Preferably, the macroscopically visible samples should be used for cell block preparation. The techniques described in this chapter can be helpful in obtaining useful and accurate specimens. Most importantly, the samples should be delivered to the Cytopathology laboratory in saline as rapidly as possible to maintain their structure without cellular degradation. It is also most important to maintain contact and communication between the urologist and cytopathologist.

Conclusion

Although upper tract urothelial carcinoma is a rare malignancy, it is potentially lethal. Urinary markers may be helpful but improvement is needed before they can become a reliable modality for diagnosis. Ureteroscopic inspection and biopsy is an essential part of the evaluation of a filling defect or other suspicion of UTUC. The introduction of ureteroscopic treatment of upper tract tumor offers a nephron-sparing option in many patients. Accurate identification of the appropriate patient relies on adequate biopsy and careful specimen preparation. Extended imaging techniques may offer improved visualization and detection of urothelial lesions.

References

1. Munoz JJ, Ellison LM. Upper tract urothelial neoplasms: incidence and survival during the last 2 decades. J Urol. 2000;164(5):1523–5.
2. Flanigan RC. Urothelial tumors of the upper urinary tract. In: Campbell-Walsh urology. 9th ed. Philadelphia: Saunders Elsevier; 2007.
3. Azemar MD, Comperat E, Richard F, Cussenot O, Roupret M. Bladder recurrence after surgery for upper urinary tract urothelial cell carcinoma: frequency, risk factors, and surveillance. Urol Oncol. 2011;29(2):130–6.
4. Feifer AH, Steinberg J, Tanguay S, Aprikian AG, Brimo F, Kassouf W. Utility of urine cytology in the workup of asymptomatic microscopic hematuria in low-risk patients. Urology. 2010;75(6):1278–82.
5. Inman BA, Tran VT, Fradet Y, Lacombe L. Carcinoma of the upper urinary tract: predictors of survival and competing causes of mortality. Cancer. 2009;115(13):2853–62.
6. McLaughlin JK, Silverman DT, Hsing AW, Ross RK, Schoenberg JB, Yu MC, Stemhagen A, Lynch CF, Blot WJ, Fraumeni Jr JF. Cigarette smoking and cancers of the renal pelvis and ureter. Cancer Res. 1992;52(2):254–7.
7. Ross RK, Paganini-Hill A, Landolph J, Gerkins V, Henderson BE. Analgesics, cigarette smoking, and other risk factors for cancer of the renal pelvis and ureter. Cancer Res. 1989;49(4):1045–8.
8. Jensen OM, Knudsen JB, McLaughlin JK, Sorensen BL. The Copenhagen case-control study of renal pelvis and ureter cancer: role of smoking and occupational exposures. Int J Cancer. 1988;41(4):557–61.
9. Hall MC, Womack S, Sagalowsky AI, Carmody T, Erickstad MD, Roehrborn CG. Prognostic factors, recurrence, and survival in transitional cell carcinoma of the upper urinary tract: a 30-year experience in 252 patients. Urology. 1998;52(4):594–601.
10. Raman JD, Shariat SF, Karakiewicz PI, Lotan Y, Sagalowsky AI, Roscigno M, Montorsi F, Bolenz C, Weizer AZ, Wheat JC, et al. Does preoperative symptom classification impact prognosis in patients with clinically localized upper-tract urothelial carcinoma managed by radical nephroureterectomy? Urol Oncol. 2011;29(6):716–23.
11. Roupret M, Zigeuner R, Palou J, Boehle A, Kaasinen E, Sylvester R, Babjuk M, Oosterlinck W. European guidelines for the diagnosis and management of upper urinary tract urothelial cell carcinomas: 2011 update. Eur Urol. 2011;59(4):584–94.
12. Olgac S, Mazumdar M, Dalbagni G, Reuter VE. Urothelial carcinoma of the renal pelvis: a clinicopathologic study of 130 cases. Am J Surg Pathol. 2004;28(12):1545–52.
13. Margulis V, Shariat SF, Matin SF, Kamat AM, Zigeuner R, Kikuchi E, Lotan Y, Weizer A, Raman JD, Wood CG, et al. Outcomes of radical nephroureterectomy: a series from the Upper Tract Urothelial Carcinoma Collaboration. Cancer. 2009;115(6):1224–33.

14. Lane BR, Smith AK, Larson BT, Gong MC, Campbell SC, Raghavan D, Dreicer R, Hansel DE, Stephenson AJ. Chronic kidney disease after nephroureterectomy for upper tract urothelial carcinoma and implications for the administration of perioperative chemotherapy. Cancer. 2010;116(12):2967–73.

15. Gadzinski AJ, Roberts WW, Faerber GJ, Wolf Jr JS. Long-term outcomes of nephroureterectomy versus endoscopic management for upper tract urothelial carcinoma. J Urol. 2010;183(6):2148–53.

16. Roupret M, Hupertan V, Traxer O, Loison G, Chartier-Kastler E, Conort P, Bitker MO, Gattegno B, Richard F, Cussenot O. Comparison of open nephroureterectomy and ureteroscopic and percutaneous management of upper urinary tract transitional cell carcinoma. Urology. 2006;67(6):1181–7.

17. Lucas SM, Svatek RS, Olgin G, Arriaga Y, Kabbani W, Sagalowsky AI, Lotan Y. Conservative management in selected patients with upper tract urothelial carcinoma compares favourably with early radical surgery. BJU Int. 2008;102(2):172–6.

18. Deligne E, Colombel M, Badet L, Taniere P, Rouviere O, Dubernard JM, Lezrek M, Gelet A, Martin X. Conservative management of upper urinary tract tumors. Eur Urol. 2002;42(1):43–8.

19. Sowter SJ, Ilie CP, Efthimiou I, Tolley DA. Endourologic management of patients with upper-tract transitional-cell carcinoma: long-term follow-up in a single center. J Endourol. 2007;21(9):1005–9.

20. Krambeck AE, Thompson RH, Lohse CM, Patterson DE, Elliott DS, Blute ML. Imperative indications for conservative management of upper tract transitional cell carcinoma. J Urol. 2007;178(3 Pt 1):792–6; discussion 796–7.

21. Roupret M, Traxer O, Tligui M, Conort P, Chartier-Kastler E, Richard F, Cussenot O. Upper urinary tract transitional cell carcinoma: recurrence rate after percutaneous endoscopic resection. Eur Urol. 2007;51(3):709–13; discussion 714.

22. Elliott DS, Segura JW, Lightner D, Patterson DE, Blute ML. Is nephroureterectomy necessary in all cases of upper tract transitional cell carcinoma? Long-term results of conservative endourologic management of upper tract transitional cell carcinoma in individuals with a normal contralateral kidney. Urology. 2001;58(2):174–8.

23. Chen GL, Bagley DH. Ureteroscopic management of upper tract transitional cell carcinoma in patients with normal contralateral kidneys. J Urol. 2000;164(4):1173–6.

24. Pak RW, Moskowitz EJ, Bagley DH. What is the cost of maintaining a kidney in upper-tract transitional-cell carcinoma? An objective analysis of cost and survival. J Endourol. 2009;23(3):341–6.

25. Wen CP, Cheng TY, Tsai MK, Chang YC, Chan HT, Tsai SP, Chiang PH, Hsu CC, Sung PK, Hsu YH, et al. All-cause mortality attributable to chronic kidney disease: a prospective cohort study based on 462 293 adults in Taiwan. Lancet. 2008;371(9631):2173–82.

26. Weiner DE, Tighiouart H, Amin MG, Stark PC, MacLeod B, Griffith JL, Salem DN, Levey AS, Sarnak MJ. Chronic kidney disease as a risk factor for cardiovascular disease and all-cause mortality: a pooled analysis of community-based studies. J Am Soc Nephrol. 2004;15(5):1307–15.

27. Go AS, Chertow GM, Fan D, McCulloch CE, Hsu CY. Chronic kidney disease and the risks of death, cardiovascular events, and hospitalization. N Engl J Med. 2004;351(13):1296–305.

28. Campbell SC, Novick AC, Belldegrun A, Blute ML, Chow GK, Derweesh IH, Faraday MM, Kaouk JH, Leveillee RJ, Matin SF, et al. Guideline for management of the clinical T1 renal mass. J Urol. 2009;182(4):1271–9.

29. McKiernan J, Simmons R, Katz J, Russo P. Natural history of chronic renal insufficiency after partial and radical nephrectomy. Urology. 2002;59(6):816–20.

30. Thompson RH, Boorjian SA, Lohse CM, Leibovich BC, Kwon ED, Cheville JC, Blute ML. Radical nephrectomy for pT1a renal masses may be associated with decreased overall survival compared with partial nephrectomy. J Urol. 2008;179(2):468–71; discussion 472–3.

31. Van Der Molen AJ, Cowan NC, Mueller-Lisse UG, Nolte-Ernsting CC, Takahashi S, Cohan RH, CT Urography Working Group of the European Society of Urogenital Radiology (ESUR). CT urography: definition, indications and techniques. A guideline for clinical practice. Eur Radiol. 2008;18(1):4–17.

32. Dillman JR, Caoili EM, Cohan RH, Ellis JH, Francis IR, Schipper MJ. Detection of upper tract urothelial neoplasms: sensitivity of axial, coronal reformatted, and curved-planar reformatted image-types utilizing 16-row multi-detector CT urography. Abdom Imaging. 2008;33(6):707–16.

33. Wang LJ, Wong YC, Chuang CK, Huang CC, Pang ST. Diagnostic accuracy of transitional cell carcinoma on multidetector computerized tomography urography in patients with gross hematuria. J Urol. 2009;181(2):524–31; discussion 531.

34. Wang LJ, Wong YC, Huang CC, Wu CH, Hung SC, Chen HW. Multidetector computerized tomography urography is more accurate than excretory urography for diagnosing transitional cell carcinoma of the upper urinary tract in adults with hematuria. J Urol. 2010;183(1):48–55.

35. Wang LJ, Wong YC, Ng KF, Chuang CK, Lee SY, Wan YL. Tumor characteristics of urothelial carcinoma on multidetector computerized tomography urography. J Urol. 2010;183(6):2154–60.

36. Ito Y, Kikuchi E, Tanaka N, Miyajima A, Mikami S, Jinzaki M, Oya M. Preoperative hydronephrosis grade independently predicts worse pathological outcomes in patients undergoing nephroureterectomy for upper tract urothelial carcinoma. J Urol. 2011;185(5):1621–6.

37. Takahashi N, Glockner JF, Hartman RP, King BF, Leibovich BC, Stanley DW, Fitz-Gibbon PD, Kawashima A. Gadolinium enhanced magnetic

resonance urography for upper urinary tract malignancy. J Urol. 2010;183(4):1330–65.

38. Takahashi N, Kawashima A, Glockner JF, Hartman RP, Leibovich BC, Brau AC, Beatty PJ, King BF. Small (<2-cm) upper-tract urothelial carcinoma: evaluation with gadolinium-enhanced three-dimensional spoiled gradient-recalled echo MR urography. Radiology. 2008;247(2):451–7.

39. Natalin RA, Prince MR, Grossman ME, Silvers D, Landman J. Contemporary applications and limitations of magnetic resonance imaging contrast materials. J Urol. 2010;183(1):27–33.

40. Brien JC, Shariat SF, Herman MP, Ng CK, Scherr DS, Scoll B, Uzzo RG, Wille M, Eggener SE, Terrell JD, et al. Preoperative hydronephrosis, ureteroscopic biopsy grade and urinary cytology can improve prediction of advanced upper tract urothelial carcinoma. J Urol. 2010;184(1):69–73.

41. Amirian MJ, Radadia K, Narins H, Healy KA, Hubosky SG, Bagley DH, Trabulsi EJ, Lallas CD. The significance of functional renal obstruction in predicting pathologic stage of upper tract urothelial carcinoma. J Endourol. 2014;28(11):1379–83.

42. El-Hakim A, Weiss GH, Lee BR, Smith AD. Correlation of ureteroscopic appearance with histologic grade of upper tract transitional cell carcinoma. Urology. 2004;63(4):647–50; discussion 650.

43. Thompson RH, Krambeck AE, Lohse CM, Elliott DS, Patterson DE, Blute ML. Endoscopic management of upper tract transitional cell carcinoma in patients with normal contralateral kidneys. Urology. 2008;71(4):713–7.

44. Keeley Jr FX, Bibbo M, Bagley DH. Ureteroscopic treatment and surveillance of upper urinary tract transitional cell carcinoma. J Urol. 1997;157(5):1560–5.

45. Keeley FX, Kulp DA, Bibbo M, McCue PA, Bagley DH. Diagnostic accuracy of ureteroscopic biopsy in upper tract transitional cell carcinoma. J Urol. 1997;157(1):33–7.

46. Williams SK, Denton KJ, Minervini A, Oxley J, Khastigir J, Timoney AG, Keeley Jr FX. Correlation of upper-tract cytology, retrograde pyelography, ureteroscopic appearance, and ureteroscopic biopsy with histologic examination of upper-tract transitional cell carcinoma. J Endourol. 2008;22(1):71–6.

47. Lotan Y, Roehrborn CG. Sensitivity and specificity of commonly available bladder tumor markers versus cytology: results of a comprehensive literature review and meta-analyses. Urology. 2003;61(1):109–18; discussion 118.

48. Rife CC, Farrow GM, Utz DC. Urine cytology of transitional cell neoplasms. Urol Clin North Am. 1979;6(3):599–612.

49. Bibbo M, Gill WB, Harris MJ, Thomsen S, Wied GL. Retrograde brushing as a diagnostic procedure of ureteral, renal pelvic and renal calyceal lesions. A preliminary report. Acta Cytol. 1974;18(2):137–41.

50. Konety BR, Getzenberg RH. Urine based markers of urological malignancy. J Urol. 2001;165(2):600–11.

51. van Rhijn BW, van der Poel HG, van der Kwast TH. Urine markers for bladder cancer surveillance: a systematic review. Eur Urol. 2005;47(6):736–48.

52. Fradet Y, Lockhard C. Performance characteristics of a new monoclonal antibody test for bladder cancer: ImmunoCyt trade mark. Can J Urol. 1997;4(3):400–5.

53. Mian C, Pycha A, Wiener H, Haitel A, Lodde M, Marberger M. Immunocyt: a new tool for detecting transitional cell cancer of the urinary tract. J Urol. 1999;161(5):1486–9.

54. Lodde M, Mian C, Wiener H, Haitel A, Pycha A, Marberger M. Detection of upper urinary tract transitional cell carcinoma with ImmunoCyt: a preliminary report. Urology. 2001;58(3):362–6.

55. Jovanovic M, Soldatovic I, Janjic A, Vuksanovic A, Dzamic Z, Acimovic M, Hadzi-Djokic J. Diagnostic value of the nuclear matrix protein 22 test and urine cytology in upper tract urothelial tumors. Urol Int. 2011;87(2):134–7.

56. Zimmerman RL, Bagley D, Hawthorne C, Bibbo M. Utility of the Bard BTA test in detecting upper urinary tract transitional cell carcinoma. Urology. 1998;51(6):956–8.

57. Ianari A, Sternberg CN, Rossetti A, Van Rijn A, Deidda A, Giannarelli D, Pansadoro V. Results of Bard BTA test in monitoring patients with a history of transitional cell cancer of the bladder. Urology. 1997;49(5):786–9.

58. Conn IG, Crocker J, Wallace DM, Hughes MA, Hilton CJ. Basement membranes in urothelial carcinoma. Br J Urol. 1987;60(6):536–42.

59. Walsh IK, Keane PF, Ishak LM, Flessland KA. The BTA stat test: a tumor marker for the detection of upper tract transitional cell carcinoma. Urology. 2001;58(4):532–5.

60. Siemens DR, Morales A, Johnston B, Emerson L. A comparative analysis of rapid urine tests for the diagnosis of upper urinary tract malignancy. Can J Urol. 2003;10(1):1754–8.

61. Schmetter BS, Habicht KK, Lamm DL, Morales A, Bander NH, Grossman HB, Hanna Jr MG, Silberman SR, Butman BT. A multicenter trial evaluation of the fibrin/fibrinogen degradation products test for detection and monitoring of bladder cancer. J Urol. 1997;158(3 Pt 1):801–5.

62. McCabe RP, Lamm DL, Haspel MV, Pomato N, Smith KO, Thompson E, Hanna Jr MG. A diagnostic-prognostic test for bladder cancer using a monoclonal antibody-based enzyme-linked immunoassay for detection of urinary fibrin(ogen) degradation products. Cancer Res. 1984;44(12 Pt 1):5886–93.

63. Johnston B, Morales A, Emerson L, Lundie M. Rapid detection of bladder cancer: a comparative study of point of care tests. J Urol. 1997;158(6):2098–101.

64. Skacel M, Fahmy M, Brainard JA, Pettay JD, Biscotti CV, Liou LS, Procop GW, Jones JS, Ulchaker J, Zippe CD, et al. Multitarget fluorescence in situ hybridization assay detects transitional cell carcinoma in the majority of patients with bladder cancer and atypical or negative urine cytology. J Urol. 2003;169(6):2101–5.

65. Sokolova IA, Halling KC, Jenkins RB, Burkhardt HM, Meyer RG, Seelig SA, King W. The development of a multitarget, multicolor fluorescence in situ hybridization assay for the detection of urothelial carcinoma in urine. J Mol Diagn. 2000;2(3):116–23.

66. Halling KC, King W, Sokolova IA, Meyer RG, Burkhardt HM, Halling AC, Cheville JC, Sebo TJ, Ramakumar S, Stewart CS, et al. A comparison of cytology and fluorescence in situ hybridization for the detection of urothelial carcinoma. J Urol. 2000;164(5):1768–75.

67. Bubendorf L, Grilli B, Sauter G, Mihatsch MJ, Gasser TC, Dalquen P. Multiprobe FISH for enhanced detection of bladder cancer in voided urine specimens and bladder washings. Am J Clin Pathol. 2001;116(1):79–86.

68. Bollmann M, Heller H, Bankfalvi A, Griefingholt H, Bollmann R. Quantitative molecular urinary cytology by fluorescence in situ hybridization: a tool for tailoring surveillance of patients with superficial bladder cancer? BJU Int. 2005;95(9):1219–25.

69. Akkad T, Brunner A, Pallwein L, Gozzi C, Bartsch G, Mikuz G, Steiner H, Verdorfer I. Fluorescence in situ hybridization for detecting upper urinary tract tumors–a preliminary report. Urology. 2007;70(4):753–7.

70. Marin-Aguilera M, Mengual L, Ribal MJ, Musquera M, Ars E, Villavicencio H, Algaba F, Alcaraz A. Utility of fluorescence in situ hybridization as a non-invasive technique in the diagnosis of upper urinary tract urothelial carcinoma. Eur Urol. 2007;51(2):409–15; discussion 415.

71. Chen AA, Grasso M. Is there a role for FISH in the management and surveillance of patients with upper tract transitional-cell carcinoma? J Endourol. 2008;22(6):1371–4.

72. Johannes JR, Nelson E, Bibbo M, Bagley DH. Voided urine fluorescence in situ hybridization testing for upper tract urothelial carcinoma surveillance. J Urol. 2010;184(3):879–82.

73. Mian C, Mazzoleni G, Vikoler S, Martini T, Knuchel-Clark R, Zaak D, Lazica A, Roth S, Mian M, Pycha A. Fluorescence in situ hybridisation in the diagnosis of upper urinary tract tumours. Eur Urol. 2010;58(2):288–92.

74. Reynolds JP, Voss JS, Kipp BR, Karnes RJ, Nassar A, Clayton AC, Henry MR, Sebo TJ, Zhang J, Halling KC. Comparison of urine cytology and fluorescence in situ hybridization in upper urothelial tract samples. Cancer Cytopathol. 2014;122(6):459–67.

75. Wang J, Wu J, Peng L, Tu P, Li W, Liu L, Cheng W, Wang X, Zhou S, Shi S, et al. Distinguishing urothelial carcinoma in the upper urinary tract from benign diseases with hematuria using FISH. Acta Cytol. 2012;56(5):533–8.

76. Xu C, Zeng Q, Hou J, Gao L, Zhang Z, Xu W, Yang B, Sun Y. Utility of a modality combining FISH and cytology in upper tract urothelial carcinoma detection in voided urine samples of Chinese patients. Urology. 2011;77(3):636–41.

77. Luo B, Li W, Deng CH, Zheng FF, Sun XZ, Wang DH, Dai YP. Utility of fluorescence in situ hybridization in the diagnosis of upper urinary tract urothelial carcinoma. Cancer Genet Cytogenet. 2009;189(2):93–7.

78. Fernandez MI, Parikh S, Grossman HB, Katz R, Matin SF, Dinney CP, Kamat AM. The role of FISH and cytology in upper urinary tract surveillance after radical cystectomy for bladder cancer. Urol Oncol. 2012;30(6):821–4.

79. Lughezzani G, Burger M, Margulis V, Matin SF, Novara G, Roupret M, Shariat SF, Wood CG, Zigeuner R. Prognostic factors in upper urinary tract urothelial carcinomas: a comprehensive review of the current literature. Eur Urol. 2012;62(1):100–14.

80. Bagrodia A, Youssef RF, Kapur P, Darwish OM, Cannon C, Belsante MJ, Gerecci D, Sagalowsky AI, Shariat SF, Lotan Y, et al. Prospective evaluation of molecular markers for the staging and prognosis of upper tract urothelial carcinoma. Eur Urol. 2012;62(1):e27–9.

81. Krabbe LM, Bagrodia A, Lotan Y, Gayed BA, Darwish OM, Youssef RF, John G, Harrow B, Jacobs C, Gaitonde M, et al. Prospective analysis of Ki-67 as an independent predictor of oncologic outcomes in patients with high grade upper tract urothelial carcinoma. J Urol. 2014;191(1):28–34.

82. Bagley DH, Grasso 3rd M. Ureteroscopic laser treatment of upper urinary tract neoplasms. World J Urol. 2010;28(2):143–9.

83. Abdel-Razzak OM, Ehya H, Cubler-Goodman A, Bagley DH. Ureteroscopic biopsy in the upper urinary tract. Urology. 1994;44(3):451–7.

84. Tawfiek ER, Bagley DH. Upper-tract transitional cell carcinoma. Urology. 1997;50(3):321–9.

85. Hudson RG, Conlin MJ, Bagley DH. Ureteric access with flexible ureteroscopes: effect of the size of the ureteroscope. BJU Int. 2005;95(7):1043–4.

86. Johnson GB, Portela D, Grasso M. Advanced ureteroscopy: wireless and sheathless. J Endourol. 2006;20(8):552–5.

87. Kleinmann N, Healy KA, Hubosky SG, Margel D, Bibbo M, Bagley DH. Ureteroscopic biopsy of upper tract urothelial carcinoma: comparison of basket and forceps. J Endourol. 2013;27(12):1450–4.

88. Tawfiek E, Bibbo M, Bagley DH. Ureteroscopic biopsy: technique and specimen preparation. Urology. 1997;50(1):117–9.

89. Bultitude MF, Ghani KR, Horsfield C, Glass J, Chandra A, Thomas K. Improving the interpretation of ureteroscopic biopsies: use of Bouin's fixative. BJU Int. 2011;108(9):1373–5.

90. Solomides CC, Birbe RC, Nicolaou N, Bagley D, Bibbo M. Does mitosis-specific marker phosphohistone H3 help the grading of upper tract urothelial carcinomas in cell blocks? Acta Cytol. 2012;56(3):285–8.

91. Cauberg EC, de Bruin DM, Faber DJ, van Leeuwen TG, de la Rosette JJ, de Reijke TM. A new generation of optical diagnostics for bladder cancer: technology, diagnostic accuracy, and future applications. Eur Urol. 2009;56(2):287–96.

Imaging of Upper Tract Transitional Cell Carcinoma

2

Sarah L. Steenbergen and Gary Israel

2.1 Introduction

While bladder and kidney cancer are the 6th and 9th most common malignancies, transitional cell carcinoma of the pelvis and ureters is much less common. It accounts for only 2–6 % of all transitional cell carcinomas, the majority of which occur in the bladder, and accounts for only 10 % of all renal tumors [1]. Upper tract transitional cell carcinoma (UTTCC) is three times more common in men than in women and the incidence increases with age with the highest prevalence in the fifth to seventh decades of life [1]. Patients with UTTCC have a variable and nonspecific presentation, hematuria being the most common presenting symptom. However, hematuria may also be secondary to more common etiologies including renal calculi, urinary tract infection, genital infection and benign prostatic hypertrophy. In some cases, patients with UTTCC may also present with symptoms of urinary obstruction or may present with symptoms of metastatic disease. While UTTCC can be diagnosed with retrograde uretopyelography or ureteroscopy, both of these exams are invasive and require general anesthesia. Noninvasive imaging, therefore, plays a major role in the diagnosis, work up and follow up of UTTCC. Historically, intravenous pyelography was the imaging gold standard for the detection of UTTCC. However, with advancements in imaging technology, this has fallen out of favor. Today, computed tomography (CT) and magnetic resonance imaging (MR) urography are the mainstays of evaluating patients for UTTCC. This chapter will review the current radiologic imaging modalities and techniques used to evaluate for UTTCC and will explore the strengths and weakness of each. Understanding the utility and limitations of the different imaging techniques is important and should lead to improved patient care and outcomes with earlier diagnosis.

2.2 Characteristics of Upper Tract Transitional Cell Carcinoma

UTTCC most commonly arises in the extrarenal pelvis, followed by the infundibulocaliceal region (Fig. 2.1). The ureter accounts for 25 % of UTTCC, of which 60–75 % of those are found in the lower third of the ureter [1, 2] (Fig. 2.2). There is equal occurrence in the right and left kidneys with 2–4 % of cases presenting bilaterally [1, 2]. Low stage, superficial, small neoplasms with slow

S.L. Steenbergen, MD • G. Israel, MD (✉)
Diagnostic Radiology, Yale New Haven Hospital,
20 York Street, New Haven, CT 06510, USA
e-mail: Sarah.steenbergen@yale.edu;
Gary.israel@yale.edu

© Springer International Publishing Switzerland 2015
M. Grasso III, D.H. Bagley (eds.), *Upper Urinary Tract Urothelial Carcinoma*,
DOI 10.1007/978-3-319-13869-5_2

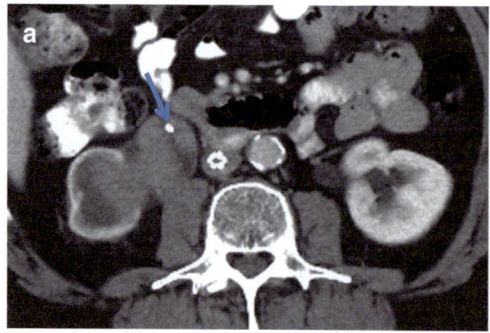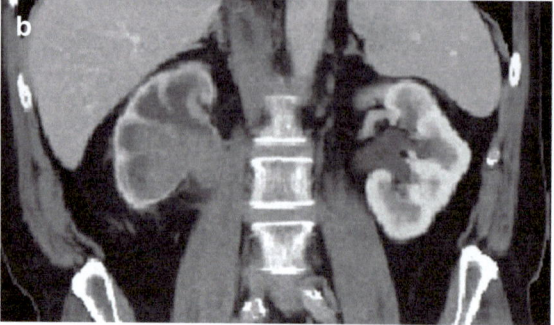

Fig. 2.1 A 64 year old male presents with right upper quadrant abdominal pain, nausea and vomiting. A right upper quadrant ultrasound (not shown) demonstrated right hydronephrosis. Axial (**a**) and coronal (**b**) contrast enhanced CT images demonstrate a mass filling and expanding the right renal pelvis. The mass extends into the right lower pole calices and down the proximal ureter resulting in hydronephrosis. This is a pathologically proven TCC. A right nephroureteral stent is in place (*arrow*)

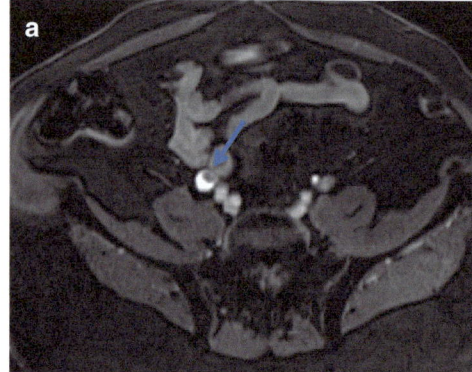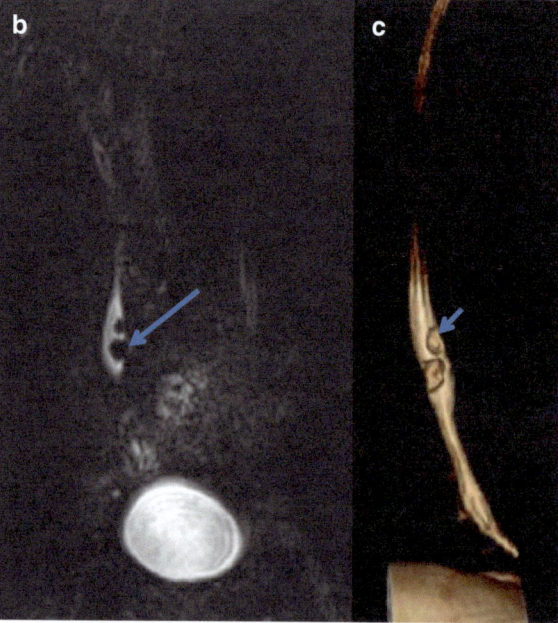

Fig. 2.2 A 62 year old male with hematuria and MR urography was performed. An axial T1-weighted fat suppressed gadolinium enhanced MR image performed 10 min after contrast administration demonstrates a filling defect (*long arrow*) in the mid right ureter (**a**). The ureteral lesion (*arrow*) is well seen on the coronal T2-weighted TSE image (**b**) and on a volume rendered 3D reformatted image (**c**). Also note a synchronous smaller lesion just cephalad to the original lesion (short *arrow* in **c**). Both lesions are pathologically proven TCC

growth and a relatively benign course account for 85 % of UTTCCs [2]. Subsequent development of metachronous UTTCC occurs in 11–13 % of patients and metachronous bladder tumors occur in 50 % of patients, typically within 2 years of treatment [2]. UTTCC can spread by mucosal extension, local invasion, hematogenously or through the lymphatic system. The most common locations for metastatic disease include lymph nodes, liver, bone and lungs [2].

2.2.1 Computed Tomography Urography

General

CT urography is currently the most commonly utilized imaging modality in the diagnosis, staging and follow up of transitional cell carcinoma [3–6]. CT urography became feasible with the advent of multidetector CT in the late 1990s, allowing for imaging of the entire abdomen and pelvis in a single breath hold with thinly collimated images. The advantages of CT include high spatial resolution, optimal detection of calcifications, and superb assessment of the kidneys, collecting system and ureters as well as the perirenal tissues and remainder of the abdomen and pelvis. The disadvantages of CT include limited contrast resolution (when compared to MRI) and exposure to iodizing radiation. CT urography also necessitates the administration of intravenous iodinated contrast, which can result in allergic reactions or renal failure. In addition, CT urography relies on contrast excretion into the collecting systems. In patients with ureteral obstruction, contrast excretion may be inhibited, impeding adequate evaluation of the collecting system and ureter.

CT urography has a sensitivity of 96 % and a specificity of 99 % for lesions 5–10 mm in size with a drop in sensitivity to 89 % for lesions less than 5 mm and to 40 % for lesions less than 3 mm in size according to the European guidelines for UTTCC [3]. A recent meta-analysis of published literature reports CT urography to have a pooled sensitivity of 96 % and a pooled specificity of 99 % for the detection of UTTCC in patients presenting with hematuria [4, 6]. Given this favorable data, the American Board of Radiology and The American Urological Association Best Practices Policy guidelines recommend CT urography as the most appropriate initial imaging test for the evaluation of asymptomatic hematuria [5].

Techniques

CT urography involves multiphasic helical imaging of the abdomen and pelvis without and with intravenous contrast. The pre-contrast scan is ideal to evaluate for renal, ureteral or bladder stones and serves as a baseline to assess for enhancement in a renal mass, if one is present. For the post-contrast portion of the exam, the American College of Radiology recommends administering 100–150 cc of 300–350 mg/ml non ionic intravenous contrast at a rate of 2–4 ml/s for the average sized adult [7]. There are a variety of methods of performing the post-contrast portion of the CT urography exam. A single bolus technique may be employed which consists of a single bolus of intravenous contrast (after the initial non-contrast images are obtained) followed by imaging of the kidneys during the nephrographic phase of enhancement (90–100 s post contrast injection) and a second post-contrast acquisition of the abdomen and pelvis during the excretory phase (5–15 min post contrast injection) [5]. The nephrogenic phase results in a homogenous nephrogram and is considered the best phase of enhancement to identify and characterize renal masses. Excretory phase imaging is used for assessing the collecting systems, ureters and bladder for non calcified filling defects, including TCC (Fig. 2.3). Overall, the single bolus CT urography technique results in a relatively high radiation exposure, equivalent to approximately 3 CT scans of the abdomen and 2 CT scans of the pelvis. Alternatively there are a variety of split bolus contrast techniques. In general, these consist of an unenhanced scan of the abdomen and pelvis followed by two reduced doses of intravenous contrast separated by 8–15 min (depending on the protocol) and with a single post contrast acquisition. The split bolus technique results in a combined nephrographic and excretory phase of enhancement which allows a single post-contrast acquisition. The advantage of this is a slightly reduced radiation dose corresponding to the elimination of one of the CT scans of the abdomen (the nephrographic phase in the single bolus technique). A disadvantage of the split bolus technique is that the contrast bolus is split, and therefore the combined nephrographic/excretory phase may not be equivalent to acquiring separate nephrographic and excretory phases.

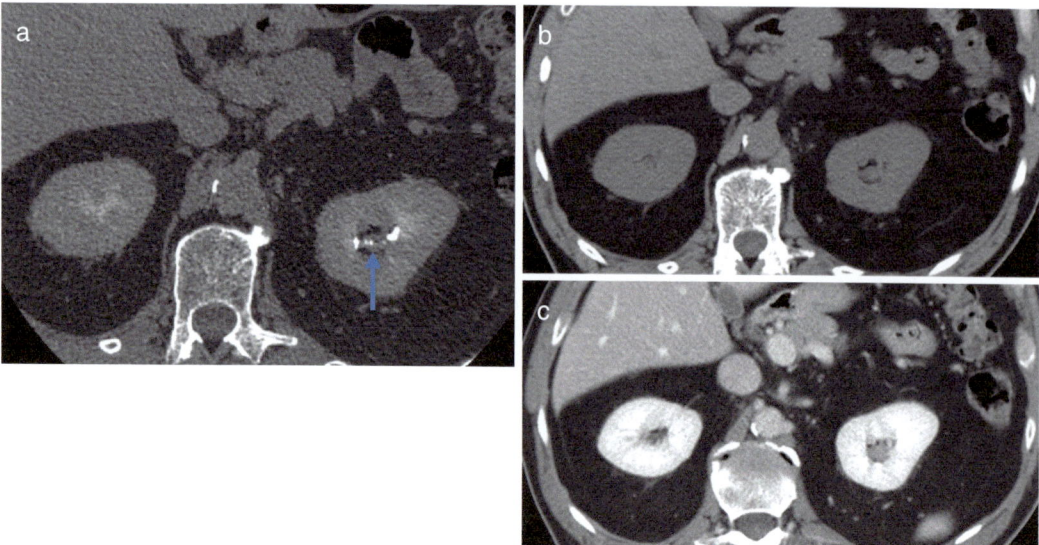

Fig. 2.3 A 61 year old male with a history of hematuria. Axial contrast enhanced CT image obtained during the excretory phase (**a**) demonstrates subtle thickening of the left upper pole infundibulum (*arrow*) which is a proven TCC. On the axial unenhanced (**b**) and contrast enhanced (**c**) CT images the mass is very difficult to detect. This case demonstrates the utility of excretory phase imaging in detecting UTTCC

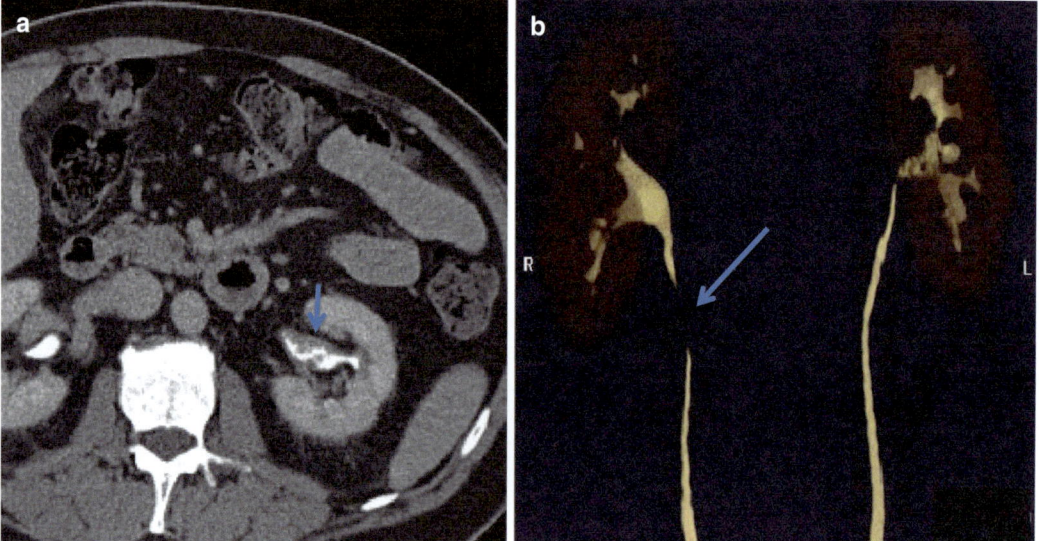

Fig. 2.4 A 56 year old male presents with hematuria. (**a**) Axial image from a CT urogram in the excretory phase demonstrates the utility of delayed contrast imaging to elucidate a transitional cell carcinoma presenting as nodular urothelial wall thickening (*short arrow*). (**b**) A volume rendered 3D image shows the irregular narrowing of the left renal pelvis. The discontinuity of the right ureter is due to poor opacification of the ureter with contrast secondary to peristalsis and is important not to mistake for disease (*long arrow*)

A shortcoming of CT urography is incomplete distention and opacification of the ureters secondary to ureteral peristalsis (Fig. 2.4). A few techniques have been evaluated to improve opacification of the ureters including supplementation with intravenous saline and/or intravenous furosemide. In one study, the addition of 10 mg intravenous furosemide given over 1 min helped opacify and distend the collecting system and ureters better than 250 cc intravenous saline alone. The study also demonstrated no additional benefit of combining furosemide with saline [8].

At Yale New Haven Hospital, we perform CT urography using a single bolus three phase (noncontrast, nephrogenic phase and excretory phase) technique in patients over 40 years of age and use a split bolus dual phase protocol (noncontast and combined nephrogenic/excretory phase) in patients under 40 years of age. Three-dimensional post-processing techniques including maximum intensity projections (MIPs) and three-dimensional reformation are helpful in evaluating the collecting systems in the coronal or oblique planes, can demonstrate the relationship between multiple lesions and provides urologists with a familiar imaging format (Figs. 2.2c and 2.4b).

Imaging Findings

TCC can have many different appearances on CT imaging. Most commonly, TCC appears as an enhancing soft tissue mass within the collecting system or ureter [6] (Figs. 2.1 and 2.2). This may obstruct a portion of the collecting system or ureter proximal to the tumor. On precontrast images, TCC is typically slightly hyperdense with respect to urine. On post contrast images TCC often demonstrates early enhancement with subsequent washout on delayed images. TCC can be seen as a sessile (Fig. 2.5) or pendunculated filling defect, a mass infiltrating the wall of the collecting system/ureter which would cause pelvicaliceal irregularity (Fig. 2.4), or circumferential thickening of the collecting system/ureter (Fig. 2.6) which can obstruct the urinary system proximally. In the ureter, the distal ureter is the most common site of TCC, accounting for 73 % of all ureteral TCCs; 24 % occur in the mid ureter (Fig. 2.2) and only 3 % in the proximal ureter [6]. Eighty-five percent of UTTCCs are small, low

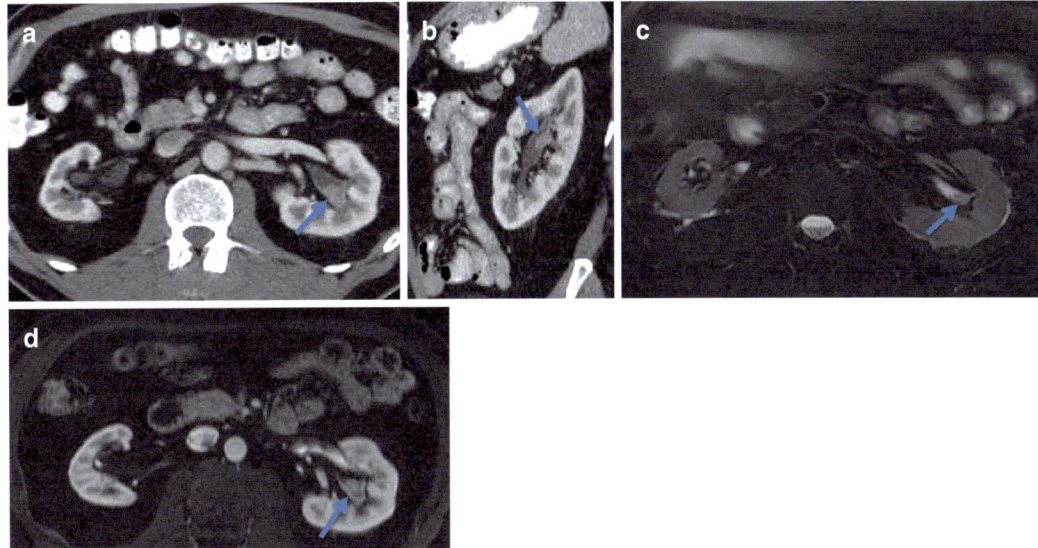

Fig. 2.5 A 58 year old male presented with 6 months of abdominal pain and right flank pain. Contrast enhanced CT in axial (**a**) and sagittal planes (**b**) shows a hyperdense filling defect (*arrow*) in the left upper pole collecting system at the infundibular-caliceal junction which was biopsied and proven to be TCC. (**c**) Axial T2-weighted fat saturation image shows the tumor as a filling defect (*arrow*) against the urine which is hyperintense in signal. (**d**) Axial contrast enhanced fat suppressed T1 weighted MR image shows that the mass (*arrow*) enhances with contrast, compatible with neoplasm

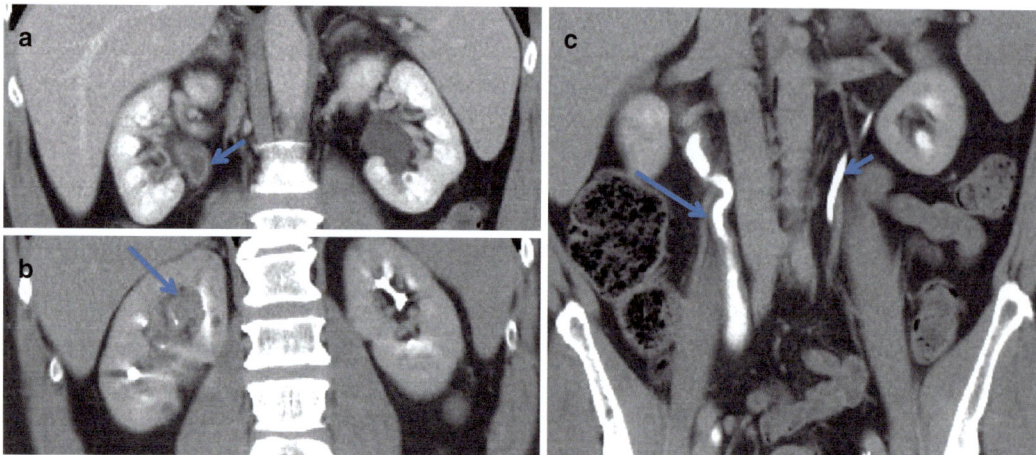

Fig. 2.6 A 55 year old male presents with hematuria after radical cystoprostatectomy and orthotopic neobladder for transitional cell carcinoma of the bladder and prosthatic urethra. Contrast enhanced CT in the coronal plane obtained during the nephrographic phase of enhancement demonstrates urothelial thickening and enhancement of the right renal pelvis (*arrow*) and proximal ureter (**a**). An excretory phase image from the same study shows a mass (*arrow*) in the infundibulocaliceal region of the upper pole which displaces the contrast in the collecting system (**b**). This mass was biopsied and confirmed to represent TCC. Disease extends inferiorly down the ureter which is markedly thickened (*long arrow*) compared to the normal left ureter (*short arrow*) (**c**)

stage, superficial, papillary neoplasms with a broad base and relatively benign course. Approximately 15 % are diffusely infiltrating tumors and these malignancies tend to present as large masses and have a more aggressive course (Fig. 2.7) [2, 9]. These extend in the renal parenchyma in an infiltrating pattern resulting in distortion of normal renal architecture.

Staging

In addition to diagnosing TCC, CT urography can be used to stage the tumor simultaneously. The overall accuracy of predicting pathologic stage with CT is 36–83 % [2]. CT allows for concurrent evaluation of the most common locations for TCC metastases, which include lymph nodes, liver, bones and lungs [2].

2.2.2 Magnetic Resonance Imaging Urography

MR urography is becoming more frequently used in the staging and surveillance of transitional cell carcinoma but it is usually only used as a first line test in the workup of symptomatic patients when CT is contraindicated. As with CT, MRI can assess for multiple possible etiologies for the patients symptoms and can evaluate the ureters, renal parenchyma, perinephric tissues and distant anatomy. While MRI has the benefit of not delivering radiation, it is more time consuming, costly and has decreased spatial resolution compared to CT urography. Furthermore, the increased acquisition time predisposes images to motion artifacts from breathing and bowel/ureter peristalsis. MR is also limited in the detection of calcifications including ureteral calculi, a common cause of hematuria that is easily detected on CT.

Gadolinium enhanced MRI can be performed on patients without concern for contrast induced nephrotoxicity and is well tolerated by patients with a history of iodinated-contrast induced allergy. The superior safety profile of gadolinium makes MRI a more appealing modality for evaluating the genitourinary system in patients who have renal disease or who have undergone nephrectomy or partial nephrectomy. Since TCC is nearly isointense to renal parenchyma on both T1 and T2 weighted images, gadolinium administration is generally suggested for evaluation of UTTCC.

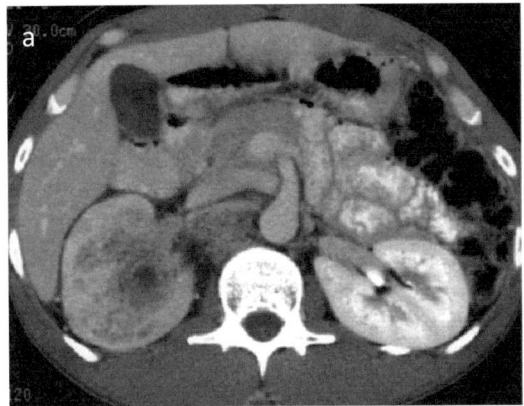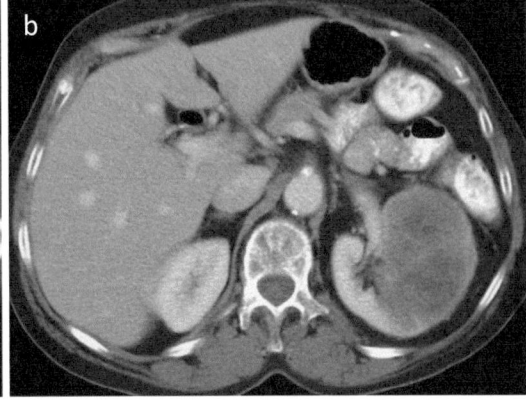

Fig. 2.7 Two different patients with infiltrative TCC of the kidney. (**a**) Axial contrast enhanced CT image demonstrates an infiltrating mass in the right kidney. Central hypodensity suggests necrosis, an aggressive feature often seen in this type of transitional cell cancer. (**b**) Axial con- trast enhanced CT image demonstrates an infiltrative mass in the left kidney which is a biopsy proven transitional cell carcinoma. Note how the reniform shape of the kidney is preserved in both cases, a finding that is not typical of renal cell carcinoma

Initial pre-contrast imaging for MR urography includes axial breath-hold T1-weighted gradient-echo (performed in and out of phase), coronal or axial breath-hold T2-weighted single-shot fast spin echo, and breath hold frequency selective fat-suppressed 3D T1-weighted spoiled gradient echo sequences. After administration of intravenous gadolinium 3D fat-suppressed T1-weighted spoiled gradient echo sequences may be performed at multiple time points and may be used to produce MR angiographic, venous, parenchymal and excretory phase images. The excretory phase of the examination is a sequence performed 5–8 min after adminis-tration of intravenous gadolinium contrast. Similar to CT, intravenous furosemide can be given at the time of gadolinium injection to aug-ment diuresis [10]. Gadolinium enhanced MR urography relies on visualization of the excreted contrast in the urine, and is therefore partially dependent on renal function. As a result, gado-linium enhanced MR urography not only pro-vides morphologic information about the kidneys, but it may also provide functional information. In patients with obstructive uropathy (in which case it may take several hours to excrete adequate amounts of contrast to fill the obstructed urinary tract), T2 weighted single shot turbo spin-echo (TSE) and 3D T2 weighted sequences can be used for MR urography. With this technique, gadolinium injection is not necessary as the fluid (urine) within the urinary tract serves as an intrin-sic contrast agent and is depicted as hyperintense on T2-weighted images (Figs. 2.5c and 2.8). This is especially useful in patients who have hydro-ureteronephrosis where a TCC may be seen as a low signal filling defect in the background of the high signal intensity urine.

Some studies comparing MR to CT in the evaluation of TCC have shown MRI to be better at tumor detection and staging although the dif-ference is not statistically significant [11]. Although MRI has superior intrinsic contrast compared to CT, the decreased spatial resolution of MRI results in a sensitivity for detection of small urothelial carcinomas under 2 cm of 74 % whereas CT has a sensitivity of 96 % [3, 9, 12]. In one study when larger lesions were included the sensitivity increased to 78 % [12]. When UTTCC results in obstruction, MR urography demon-strates an accuracy rate of 88 % or higher [13]. One recent study demonstrated utility in adding diffusion-weighted sequences for the evaluation of UTTCC. They found that in patients with a negative urine cytology the addition of diffusion-weighted imaging had both a positive predictive value and negative predictive value greater than 90 % for the detection of upper urinary tract

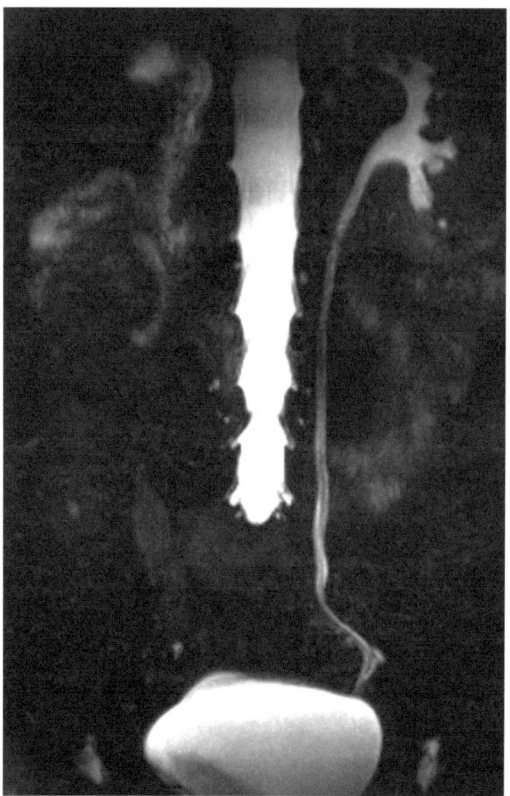

Fig. 2.8 A 51 year old female status post right nephro-ureterectomy for transitional cell carcinoma. This 3D T2-weighted turbo spin echo (TSE) maximum intensity projection (MIP) image shows a normal left collecting system. This technique takes advantage of the intrinsic high signal of urine on this sequence and can be useful in patients with poor renal function who do not excrete contrast material or in those with obstructive uropathy

cancer [14]. To the best of our knowledge, there are no studies to date directly comparing CT urography with MR urography for the detection and evaluation of UTTCC.

2.2.3 Positron Emission Tomography

18F-FDG PET/CT is a commonly used modality for staging and surveillance of multiple malignancies. 18F-FDG is excreted by the collecting system and therefore the evaluation of a collecting system malignancy can be easily obscured by normal intense accumulation of tracer in the

urinary tract. Currently, the evaluation of UTTCC with PET is limited and the major utility of PET is determining nodal involvement and distant metastases [15]. Since PET relies on metabolic activity it has the potential to detect metastatic disease in small lymph nodes. The sensitivity and specificity for detecting metastatic disease is therefore greater with PET compared to CT [15]. The sensitivity and specificity of PET/CT in the evaluation of nodal disease, regional disease and distant metastases in untreated patients with TCC is 77 % and 97 % respectively [16]. However, the sensitivity drops to as low as 50 % in patients who have previously received chemotherapy. This is likely due to decreased metabolic activity of tumor after treatment.

Conclusion

Radiology plays a major role in the diagnosis, work up and follow up of upper tract transitional cell carcinoma (UTTCC). The greatest factor in determining the most appropriate management of TCC is early detection and accurate staging. Understanding the strengths and weaknesses of the different imaging modalities available today will hopefully lead to earlier diagnosis, better staging and improved patient outcomes. It is expected that as new ways to image patients with UTTCC are developed and tested, our approach to evaluating these patients will be modified.

References

1. Lerner SP, Schoenberg M, Sternberg C, editors. Textbook of bladder cancer. London: CRC Press; 2006. p. 237–41.
2. Browne RFJ, Meehan CP, Colville J, et al. Transitional cell carcinoma of the upper urinary tract: spectrum of imaging findings. Radiographics. 2005;25:1609–27.
3. Roupret M, Babjuk M, Comperat E, et al. European guidelines for the diagnosis and management of upper tract urothelial cell carcinomas: 2011 update. Eur Assoc Urol. 2013;63:1059–71.
4. Chlapoutakis K, Theocharopoulos N, Yarmenitis S, Damilakis J. Performance of computed tomographic urography in diagnosis of upper urinary tract urothelial carcinoma, in patients presenting with hematuria: systematic review and meta-analysis. Eur J Radiol. 2010;73(2):334–8.

5. Alderson SM, Hilton S, Papanicolaou N. CT urography: review of techniques and spectrum of diseases. Applied Radiology. 2011. http://www.appliedradiology.com/articles/ct-urography-review-of-technique-and-spectrum-of-diseases. Accessed 10 Aug 2014.

6. Vikram R, Sandler CM, Ng CS. Imaging and staging of transitional cell carcinoma: part 2. Upper Urinary Tract AJR. 2009;192:1488–93.

7. CT accreditation program clinical image quality guide. American College of Radiology. 2011. http://www.acr.org/~/media/ACR/Documents/Accreditation/CT/ImageGuide.pdf. Accessed 10 Aug 2014.

8. Silverman SG, Akbar SA, Mortele KJ, et al. Multidetector row CT urography of normal urinary collecting system: furosemide versus saline as adjunct to contrast medium. Radiology. 2006;240(3):749–55.

9. Davarpanah AH, Israel G. MR imaging of the kidneys and adrenal glands. Radiol Clin North Am. 2003;41:145–59.

10. Israel G. MRI of the kidney and urinary tract. J Magn Reson Imaging. 2006;24:725–34.

11. Kim B, Semelka RC, Ascher SM, et al. Bladder tumor staging: comparison of contrast-enhanced CT, T1- and T2- weighted MR imaging, dynamic gadolinium-enhanced imaging, and late gadolinium-enhanced imaging. Radiology. 1994;193:239–45.

12. Takahashi N, Kawashima A, Glockner J, et al. Small (<2-cm) upper-tract urothelial carcinoma: evaluation with gadolinium-enhanced three-dimensional spoiled gradient-recalled echo MR urography. Radiology. 2008;247:2.

13. Takahashi N, Kawashima A, Glockner J, et al. MR urography for suspected upper tract urothelial carcinoma. Eur Radiol. 2009;19:912–23.

14. Yoshida S, Masuda H, Ishii C, et al. Usefulness of diffusion-weighted MRI in diagnosis of upper urinary tract cancer. AJR Am J Roentgenol. 2011;196:110–6.

15. Palou J, Carrio I, Villaviciencio H. Urothelial cell carcinoma in upper urinary tract – role of PET imaging. In: Rosette J, Manyak M, Harisinghani M, Wijkstra H, editors. Imaging in oncologic urology. London: Springer; 2009. p. 155–60.

16. Patil VV, Wang ZJ, Sollitto RA, et al. 18F-FDG PET/CT of transitional cell carcinoma. Am J Roentgenol. 2009;193(6):497–504.

Cytopathology and Management of Ureteroscopic Biopsy Samples

Shuyue Ren and Marluce Bibbo

3.1   Introduction

Evaluation of ureteroscopic samples requires familiarity with the cytologic features of benign conditions as well as features of Upper Tract Urinary Carcinomas (UTUC). Urinary cytology, including voided urine, catheterized bladder urine, and aspiration of ureter and pelvis, has been established for the diagnosis and surveillance of the UTUC. It is not sensitive for the diagnosis of low grade UTUC, however, the sensitivity for the high grade tumors is higher and it depends on the experiences of pathologists, ranging from 40 to 79 % [1–8]. Since tissue specimens obtained ureteroscopically are small, techniques for handling the samples are important [9]. In the past, ureteroscopic biopsies were processed routinely as histology specimens in our pathology laboratory but many did not survive routine tissue processing. The special procedure to handle ureteroscopic

samples in the cytology laboratory at our institution, to achieve the best diagnostic results, is described below.

3.2   Sample Management

The following samples obtained during the ureteroscopic procedure are submitted fresh, that is, without fixation, to the cytology laboratory:

1. Bladder urine
2. Saline wash and aspirate from site of lesion(s)
3. Biopsy of the lesion (s) in saline
4. Post-biopsy aspirate
5. Post-laser aspirate

All samples, including biopsies, are processed in the cytology laboratory, where cytospins, ThinPreps and cell blocks are prepared.

The urine and aspirates are prepared by cytocentrifugation (Cytospin) or filtration method (ThinPrep) after fixation with alcohol 95 %. The specimen is then stained with the Papanicolaou stain.

When larger tissue fragments are visualized in the biopsy specimen, they are transferred to a fenestrated bag and wet in formalin for cell block preparation. The bag is tissue paper wrapped and placed in a tissue cassette. The tissue in the cell block is processed as a standard biopsy, that is, fixed in formalin, embedded in paraffin, sectioned

S. Ren, MD, PhD
Department of Pathology, Anatomy and Cell Biology,
Thomas Jefferson University, 132 South 10th Street,
Philadelphia, PA 19107, USA
e-mail: shuyueren@gmail.com

M. Bibbo, MD, ScD (✉)
Department of Pathology, Thomas Jefferson University,
132 South 10th Street, Suite 260 Main, Philadelphia,
PA 19107, USA
e-mail: Marluce.bibbo@jefferson.edu

© Springer International Publishing Switzerland 2015
M. Grasso III, D.H. Bagley (eds.), *Upper Urinary Tract Urothelial Carcinoma*,
DOI 10.1007/978-3-319-13869-5_3

and H&E stained. For smaller tissue fragments the cell block is prepared by centrifugation and the pellet is wrapped in tissue paper, placed in a tissue cassette and processed as described above.

Recently we introduced the Cellient method, an automated cell block preparation system for small biopsies [10]. There are a number of advantages of the Cellient process compared to other cell block techniques. Cell loss during centrifugation and decanting is minimized. There is no additional loss of material due to incomplete transfer by the histologist from the cassette to the wax mold. Due to the efficiency of the flow-through extractions and elimination of carrier substances, complete processing uses a lower volume of reagents than standard tissue processors, without microwave radiation, and has a processing time that is significantly less than a standard tissue processor. In our experience, Cellient cell block is often used for scant specimen where otherwise no traditional cell block can be obtained and therefore additional ancillary studies can be performed if necessary. When generous biopsy materials are available, traditional cell blocks are usually prepared in our laboratory.

The close cooperation between the cytology and urology staff allows for better diagnostic results. Importantly, all samples should be delivered in saline as rapidly as possible to keep the cellular preservation.

3.3 Specimen Evaluation

3.3.1 Cytologic Specimens

The cytodiagnostic categories in the interpretation of urine, washing and aspirate specimens are:

Negative for malignancy
Positive for Malignancy
  High grade urothelial carcinoma
  Low grade urothelial carcinoma
Suspicious for urothelial carcinoma
Cannot exclude malignancy
Atypical urothelial cells

The key cytologic features for low grade and high grade urothelial carcinoma are summarized below and shown in Figs. 3.1 and 3.2:

Key Features of Low Grade Urothelial Carcinoma

Umbrella cells variable
Haphazard growth pattern
Large cells
High N/C ratio
Irregular nuclear membranes
Small nucleoli
Granular chromatin
Mitoses infrequent

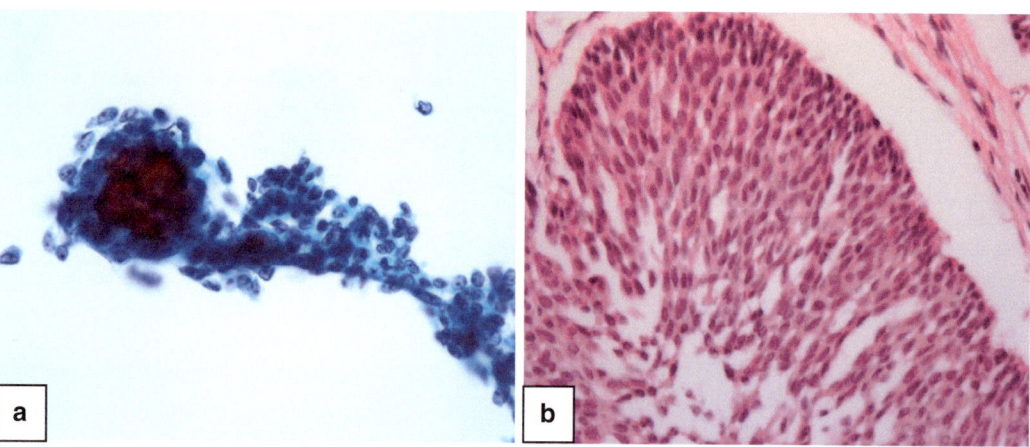

Fig. 3.1 Ureteral aspirate from a patient with a low grade papillary urothelial carcinoma of the ureter. Tumor cells have slightly enlarged and crowded nuclei. (**a**) Thinprep, Papanicolaou stain ×400. (**b**) Cell block, H&E stain ×400

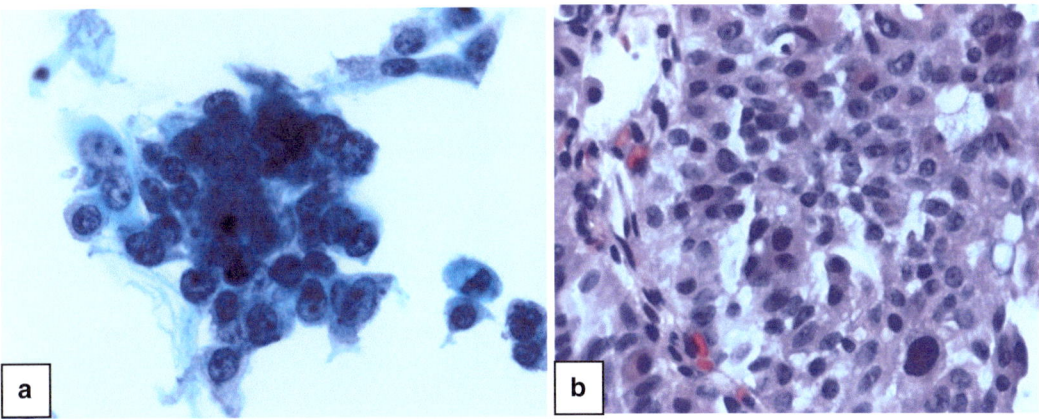

Fig. 3.2 High grade urothelial carcinoma of ureter. Note enlarged nuclei with coarse chromatin and nucleoli. (**a**) Thinprep, Papanicolau stain ×600. (**b**) Cell block, H&E stain ×600

Key Features of High Grade Urothelial Carcinoma

Absent umbrella cells
Haphazard growth pattern
Large cells
High N/C ratio
Irregular nuclear membranes
Prominent nucleoli
Coarse chromatin
Mitoses frequent
Cytoplasmic differentiation (glandular/squamous)

Caution in the interpretation of cytologic samples is necessary because specimens from the upper urinary tract contain large number of superficial cells and may show some multinucleation or atypia not seen in catheterized bladder urine cells and can be misinterpreted as malignant. Adherence to clear cut nuclear criteria of malignancy will prevent the misdiagnosis.

Post laser ureteral washings show an artifact of cellular spindling (Fig. 3.3), which occur in single cells or loose clusters and have elongated nuclei with dense chromatin. The changes are due to an epithelial response to heat.

Metastatic carcinoma to the upper urinary tract needs to be considered in the differential diagnoses, though rare, such as renal cell carcinoma (Fig. 3.4).

3.3.2 Histologic Specimens

Multiple grading schemes have been developed and employed for urinary tumors throughout the years such as the WHO 1973 classification [11, 12]. This classification includes urothelial papilloma and three grades of papillary carcinoma (grade 1, grade 2, and grade 3). This classification allows intermediate grades such as grade 1–2 and grade 2–3 to reflect tumor heterogeneity. Urothelial carcinoma grade correlates with the probability of recurrence, invasion, and metastasis, in addition to survival [13–16]. Presently we follow an adapted version of the 2004 World Health Organization (WHO) classification for UTUC [17]. This classification includes papillary urothelial neoplasm of low malignant potential (PUNLMP), low grade carcinoma and high grade carcinoma. The relationship between WHO 1973 and 2004 is shown in the Table 3.1.

At Jefferson, samples from upper urinary tract are interpreted by pathologists with experience in grading UTUC (Figs. 3.1, 3.2, 3.3 and 3.4).

Our ability to diagnose and grade UTUC has markedly improved since adopting the described sample processing in the cytology laboratory, from 40 to 90 % combining cytospin and cell block specimens [8].

There has been concern regarding ureteroscopic biopsies not reflecting the actual tumor grade. In one of our studies comparing ureteroscopic biopsies and

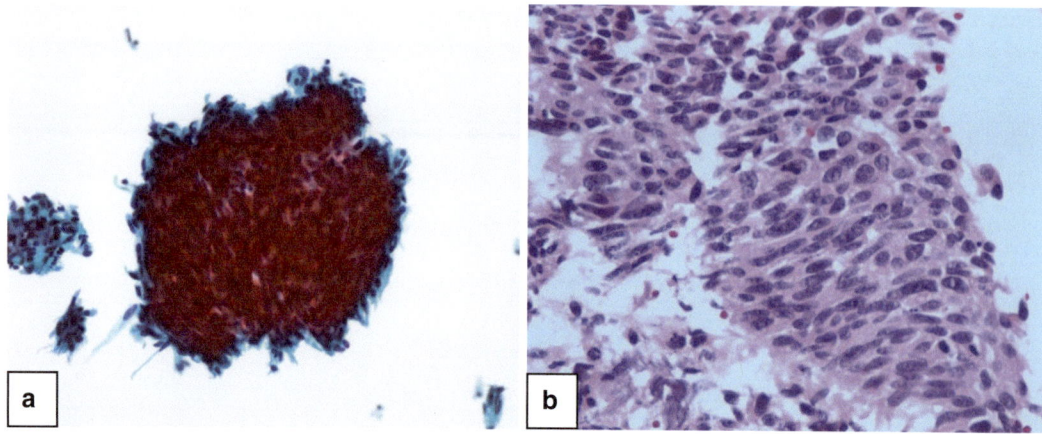

Fig. 3.3 Low grade urothelial carcinoma of the ureter after laser treatment. (**a**) Thinprep, Papanicolau stain ×200. (**b**) Cell block, H&E stain ×400

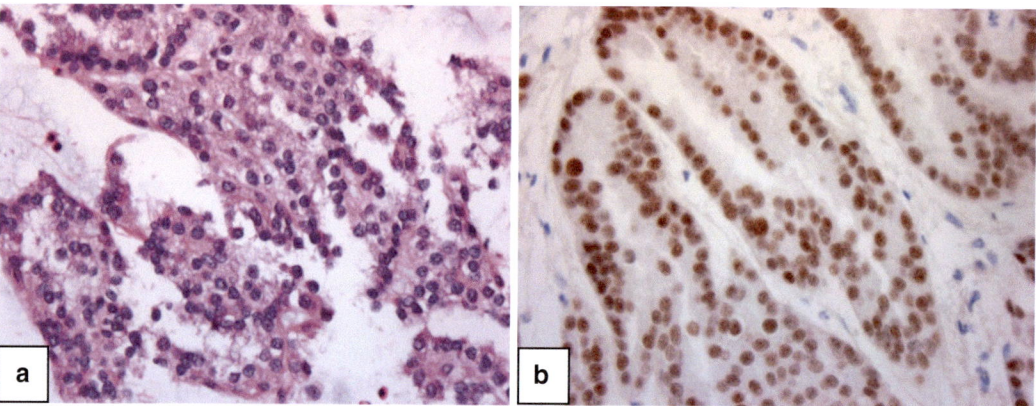

Fig. 3.4 Papillary renal cell carcinoma metastastic to the ureter. (**a**) Cell block H&E. ×400. (**b**) Pax 8 immunostain ×400 (a marker for RCC)

Table 3.1 Relationship between tumor grading systems

WHO 1973	WHO 2004
1	PUNLMP
1–2 or 2	Low grade carcinoma
2–3 or 3	High grade carcinoma

cytologic specimens with open surgical specimens of urothelial tumors, accurate information regarding grade and stage was obtained. Grading of ureteroscopic specimens was possible in 82.4 % and accurately predicted tumor grade and stage in the surgical specimens [18]. Williams et al. [19] have also demonstrated concordance between endoscopic biopsies and final pathologic specimens.

3.4 Adjunct Testing

Grading UTUC may be challenging and interobserver agreement among general pathologists is poor. Cytology alone was found to be poorly sensitive (40 %) but highly specific (79 %) for the detection of UTUC [1–8].

Fluorescence in situ hybridization (FISH) was found to increase the sensitivity of cytology and decrease specificity [20] but it also resulted in many false-positive cases. Johannes et al. [21] reported a limited value of FISH for upper tract tumor surveillance.

Some studies have investigated the prognostic impact of various biologic markers that are related to cellular processes such as cell adhesion, cell differentiation, angiogenesis, cell proliferation, epithelial mesenchymal transition, mitosis, apoptosis and vascular invasion [22, 23].

p53 is an important factor in cell cycle regulation and was found to be a predictor of UTUC patient survival in univariable analyses, it did not emerge as an independent prognostic factor after adjustment for other clinical and pathologic characteristics [24–29].

The overexpression of Ki-67, a protein involved in cell proliferation, was found to be associated with advanced tumor stage and higher grade and to be an independent predictor of survival [30].

Epidermal growth factor receptor (EGFR) is strictly related to cell growth, proliferation, and differentiation. The overexpression of EGFR was found to be associated with advanced UTUC and metaplastic differentiation but not with cancer-specific survival in multivariable analysis [31].

Several apoptosis-related markers have also been investigated in patients with UTUC. The overexpression of survivin and Bcl-2, although associated with higher tumor grade and stage, was not associated with patient survival, according to a retrospective study by Nakanishi et al. [32].

Angiogenesis is essential for human tumor growth. Increased levels of hypoxia-inducible factor 1a were found to be associated with both recurrence-free survival and cancer-specific survival by two single institutional studies, even after adjustment for several clinicopathologic variables [33, 34]. Similarly, an increased expression of metalloproteinases was shown to correlate with cancer aggressiveness and to be an independent predictor of prognosis in two studies [35, 36].

The prognostic value of molecules involved in cell adhesion was also evaluated by several investigators. A lower expression of E-cadherin was shown to be associated with higher tumor stage and grade [37]. E-cadherin was confirmed as an independent factor when predicting recurrence-free survival and cancer-specific survival [35, 38].

Microsatellite instability (MSI) is an independent molecular maker used for tumor prognosis [30]. In addition, MSI can help detect germ-line mutations, allowing for the detection of possible hereditary cancers.

Solomides et al. [39] investigated the use of a mitotic specific marker phospho-histone H3 – PHH3 as an adjunct to H&E stain for grading UTUC in cell blocks. The inter observer agreement in tumor grading improved dramatically by adding the PHH3 stain.

To date, because of the rarity of the disease, the main limitations shared by these studies are their retrospective nature and their small sample size, none of the markers has fulfilled the clinical and statistical criteria necessary to support their introduction in daily clinical decision making [23].

3.5 Concluding Remarks

Grading has become the most predictive value in defining therapy approach. The technique for specimen handling above described can be used to improve diagnostic accuracy. The accuracy of ureteroscopic biopsy and its ability to provide reliable prognostic information is important for guiding treatment of UTUC.

References

1. Renshaw AA. Comparison of ureteral washing and biopsy specimens in the community setting. Cancer. 2006;108:45–8.
2. Potts SA, Thomas PA, Cohen MB, Raab SS. Diagnostic accuracy and key cytologic features of high-grade transitional cell carcinoma in the upper urinary tract. Mod Pathol. 1997;10:657–62.
3. Boccon Gibod L, Chiche R, Dalian D, Steg A. Upper tract urothelial tumors. Diagnostic efficiency of radiology and urinary cytology. Eur Urol. 1982;8:145–7.
4. Zincke H, Aguilo JJ, Farrow GM, Utz DC, Khan AU. Significance of urinary cytology in the early detection of transitional cell cancer of the upper urinary tract. J Urol. 1976;116:781–3.
5. Skolarikos A, Griffiths TR, Powell PH, Thomas DJ, Neal DE, Kelly JD. Cytologic analysis of ureteral washings is informative in patients with grade 2 upper tract TCC considering endoscopic treatment. Urology. 2003;61:1146–50.
6. Rubben H, Hering F, Dahm HH, Lutzeyer W. Value of exfoliative urinary cytology for differentiation between uric acid stone and tumor of upper urinary tract. Urology. 1982;20:571–3.
7. Messer J, Shariat SF, Brien JC, Herman MP, Ng CK, Scherr DS, Scoll B, Uzzo RG, Wille M, Eggener SE, Steinberg G, Terrell JD, Lucas SM, Lotan Y,

Boorjian SA, Raman JD. Urinary cytology has a poor performance for predicting invasive or high-grade upper-tract urothelial carcinoma. BJU Int. 2011;108(5):701–5.

8. Chaubal A, McCue PA, Bagley DH, et al. Multimodal cytologic evaluation of upper urinary tract urothelial lesions. J Surg Pathol. 1995;1:31–5.

9. Tawfiek E, Bibbo M, Bagley DH. Ureteroscopic biopsy: technique and specimen preparation. Urology. 1997;50:117–9.

10. Wagner DG, Russell DK, Benson JM, Schneider AE, Hoda RS, Bonfiglio TA. Cellient™ automated cell block versus traditional cell block preparation: a comparison of morphologic features and immunohistochemical staining. Diagn Cytopathol. 2011;39(10):730–6.

11. Montironi R, Lopez-Beltran A, Mazzucchelli R, Bostwick DG. Classification and grading of the non-invasive urothelial neoplasms: recent advances and controversies. J Clin Pathol. 2003;56:91–5.

12. Mostofi FK, Sorbin LH, Torloni H. Histological typing of urinary bladder tumours, International classification of tumours, vol. 19. Geneva: World Health Organisation; 1973.

13. Kaubisch S, Lum BL, Reese J, et al. Stage T1 bladder cancer: grade is the primary determinant for risk of muscle invasion. J Urol. 1991;146:28–31.

14. Takashi M, Sakata T, Murase T, et al. Grade 3 bladder cancer with lamina propria invasion—pT1: characteristics of tumor and clinical course. Nagoya J Med Sci. 1991;53:1–8.

15. Thrasher JB, Frazier HA, Robertson JE, et al. Clinical variables that serve as predictors of cancer-specific survival among patients treated with radical cystectomy for transitional cell carcinoma of the bladder and prostate. Cancer. 1994;73:1708–15.

16. Torti FM, Lum BL. Superficial bladder cancer: risk of recurrence and potential role for interferon therapy. Cancer. 1987;59:613–20.

17. Eble JN, Sauter G, Epstein JI, Sesterhenn IA. Pathology and genetics of tumours of the urinary system and male genital organs, World Health Organization classification of tumours. Lyon: IARC Press; 2004. p. 10.

18. Keeley FX, Kulp DA, Bibbo M, et al. Diagnostic accuracy of ureteroscopic biopsy in upper tract transitional cell carcinoma. J Urol. 1997;157:33–7.

19. Williams S, Denton K, Minervini A, et al. Correlation of upper tract cytology, retrograde pyelography, ureteroscopic biopsy with histologic examination of upper tract transitional cell carcinoma. J Endourol. 2008;22:71–6.

20. Reynolds JP, Voss JS, Kipp BR, Karnes RJ, Nassar A, Clayton AC, Henry MR, Sebo TJ, Zhang J, Halling KC. Comparison of urine cytology and fluorescence in situ hybridization in upper urothelial tract samples. Cancer Cytopathol. 2014. doi:10.1002/cncy.21414. [Epub ahead of print].

21. Johannes JR, Nelson E, Bibbo M, Bagley DH. Voided urine fluorescence in situ hybridization testing for upper tract urothelial carcinoma surveillance. J Urol. 2010;184(3):879–82.

22. Rouprêt M, Babjuk M, Compérat E, Zigeuner R, Sylvester R, Burger M, Cowan NC, Böhle A, Van Rhijn BWG, Kaasinen E, Palou J, Shariat SF. European Guidelines on Upper Tract Urothelial Carcinomas: 2013 Update. Eur Urol. 2013;63:1059–1071.

23. Lughezzani G, Burger M, Margulis V, et al. Prognostic factors in upper urinary tract urothelial carcinomas: a comprehensive review of the current literature. Eur Urol. 2012;62(1):100–14.

24. Minimo C, Bagley DH, Bibbo M. The role of computerized quantitation of immunohistochemical staining of p53 protein in grading upper urinary tract urothelial lesions. J Urol Pathol. 1996;4:261–71.

25. Minimo C, Tawfiek ER, Bagley DH, et al. Grading of upper urinary tract transitional cell carcinomaby computed DNA content and p53 expression. Urology. 1997;50:869–74.

26. Keeley FX, Bibbo M, McCue P, et al. Use of p53 in the diagnosis of upper tract transitional cell carcinoma. Urology. 1997;49:181–6.

27. Weaver EJ, McCue PA, Bibbo M, et al. Expression of cytokeratin 20 and CD 44 protein in upper urinary tract transitional cell carcinoma. Cytologic-histologic correlation. Anal Quant Cytol Histol. 2001;23: 339–44.

28. Hashimoto H, Sue Y, Saga Y, Tokumitsu M, Yachiku S. Roles of p53 and MDM2 in tumor proliferation and determination of the prognosis of transitional cell carcinoma of the renal pelvis and ureter. Int J Urol. 2000;7:457–63.

29. Zigeuner R, Tsybrovskyy O, Ratschek M, Rehak P, Lipsky K, Langner C. Prognostic impact of p63 and p53 expression in upper urinary tract transitional cell carcinoma. Urology. 2004;63:1079–83.

30. Jeon HG, Jeong IG, Bae J, et al. Expression of Ki-67 and COX-2 in patients with upper urinary tract urothelial carcinoma. Urology. 2010;76:513. e7–12.

31. Leibl S, Zigeuner R, Hutterer G, Chromecki T, Rehak P, Langner C. EGFR expression in urothelial carcinoma of the upper urinary tract is associated with disease progression and metaplastic morphology. APMIS. 2008;116:27–32.

32. Nakanishi K, Tominaga S, Hiroi S, et al. Expression of survivin does not predict survival in patients with transitional cell carcinoma of the upper urinary tract. Virchows Arch. 2002;441:559–63.

33. Nakanishi K, Hiroi S, Tominaga S, et al. Expression of hypoxiainducible factor-1alpha protein predicts survival in patients with transitional cell carcinoma of the upper urinary tract. Clin Cancer Res. 2005;11: 2583–90.

34. Ke HL, Wei YC, Yang SF, et al. Overexpression of hypoxia-inducible factor-1alpha predicts an unfavorable outcome in urothelial carcinoma of the upper urinary tract. Int J Urol. 2008;15:200–5.

35. Inoue K, Kamada M, Slaton JW, et al. The prognostic value of angiogenesis and metastasis-related genes for progression of transitional cell carcinoma of the renal pelvis and ureter. Clin Cancer Res. 2002;8: 1863–70.

36. Miyata Y, Kanda S, Nomata K, Hayashida Y, Kanetake H. Expression of metalloproteinase-2, metalloproteinase-9, and tissue inhibitor of metallo-proteinase-1 in transitional cell carcinoma of upper urinary tract: correlation with tumor stage and sur-vival. Urology. 2004;63:602–8.

37. Nakanishi K, Kawai T, Torikata C, Aurues T, Ikeda T. E-cadherin expression in upper-urinary-tract carci-noma. Int J Cancer. 1997;74:446–9.

38. Fromont G, Rouprêt M, Amira N, et al. Tissue micro-array analysis of the prognostic value of E-cadherin, Ki67, p53, p27, survivin and MSH2 expression in upper urinary tract transitional cell carcinoma. Eur Urol. 2005;48:764–70.

39. Solomides C, Birbe R, Nicolaou N, et al. Does mitosis specific marker PHH3 help grading upper tract uro-thelial carcinomas in cell blocks? Acta Cytol. 2012;56:285–8.

Ureteropyeloscopic Treatment of Upper Urinary Tract Urothelial Malignancy

4

Michael Grasso III, Bobby S. Alexander, Lynn J. Paik, and Andrew I. Fishman

4.1 Introduction

The treatment of upper urinary tract urothelial malignancy has paralleled similar therapies in the lower urinary tract. The majority of bladder tumors that are superficial, non-invasive, and low grade in histology are treated endoscopically, not with extirpative surgery. Prohibitive factors historically with regard to treating upper tract lesions endoscopically have been the large size and poor directability of the original ureteroscopes and the limited efficacy and availability of energy sources to treat these lesions. This has evolved as endoscopic instrumentation has improved. Endoscope

miniaturization with improved mechanics have allowed for complete inspection of the entire upper urinary tract, and the application of various wavelengths of laser light energy employed to both coagulate and resect upper tract urothelial tumors have remarkably changed how these lesions are treated.

The ureteroscope has evolved from a diagnostic instrument into a therapeutic tool. The ability to not only access an upper tract urothelial lesion but to sample and then completely treat it has changed the management of this disease. In this chapter we will present the tenets of diagnostic ureteroscopy. We will then frame ureterosurgical technique to treat various upper tract urothelial lesions. Finally, we will review outcomes with regard to treating upper tract urothelial lesions of varying histology, comparing outcomes with the traditional extirpative nephroureterectomy.

4.2 Diagnostic Ureteroscopy

Bagley and his colleagues at the University of Chicago first described diagnostic ureteroscopic technique [1]. This included employing a rigid ureteroscope to evaluate and map the ureter, while an actively deflectable flexible ureteroscope was employed to asses the intra-renal collecting system. Miniaturization of the rigid instrument, based on fiberoptic imaging, allowed the now *semi-rigid* ureteroscope to be passed directly

M. Grasso III, MD (✉)
Department of Urology, New York Medical College, Valhalla, New York, USA
e-mail: mgrasso3@earthlink.net

B.S. Alexander, MD
Department of Urology, Lenox Hill Hospital, 100 E 77 Street, 4 East, New York, NY 10075, USA
e-mail: balexander23@hotmail.com

L.J. Paik, DO
Department of Urology, Lenox Hill Hospital, New York, NY 10075, USA
e-mail: ljpaik@gmail.com

A.I. Fishman, MD
Department of Urology, New York Medical College, Valhalla, NY 10595, USA
e-mail: afishman@Iupny.com

© Springer International Publishing Switzerland 2015
M. Grasso III, D.H. Bagley (eds.), *Upper Urinary Tract Urothelial Carcinoma*,
DOI 10.1007/978-3-319-13869-5_4

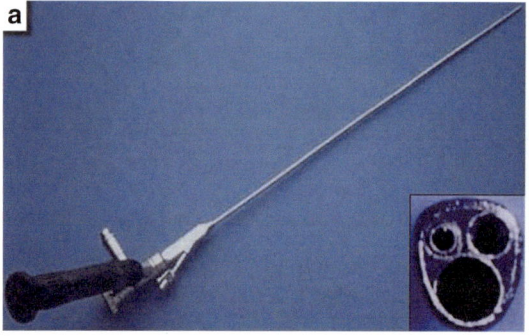
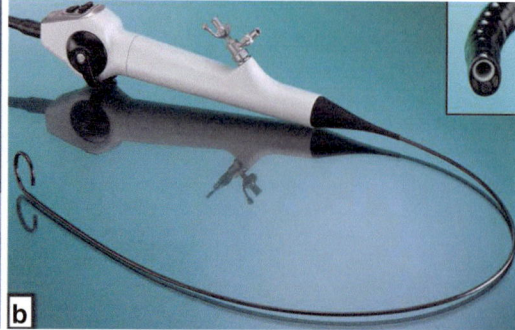

Fig. 4.1 The semirigid ureteroscope (**a**=shown is the ACMI MR6 model) can be utilized to inspect the distal ureter, while the flexible ureteroscope (**b**=shown is the Karl Storz Flex Xc digital model) allows meticulous inspection of the entire ureter and intra-renal collecting system. *Inset*: the tips of each scope reveal the lighting element, lens, and working channel

into the ureter, often without dilation or a guide-wire. The "no touch" technique minimized access trauma which could obscure a malignant lesion, or produce a false positive [2, 3]. The semi-rigid endoscope (Fig. 4.1a) is employed to inspect the distal half of the ureter, while an actively deflectable fiberoptic ureteropyeloscope (Fig. 4.1b) is employed to evaluate the proximal ureter and intra-renal collecting system. A careful systematic mapping of the upper urinary tract urothelium is essential, with each calyx and papilla inspected. Minimizing the use of retrograde catheters and guidewires minimizes hematuria intraoperatively, which can obscure the operative field. This no touch technique, where the endoscope is passed without a guidewire or an operative sheath, optimizes the surgeon's ability to differentiate a malignant lesion from ureteral wall trauma secondary to retrograde manipulation.

With smaller fiberoptic bundles for imaging, the actively deflectable flexible ureteroscope was miniaturized to an average shaft diameter of slightly larger than 8 French. The flexible endoscope could now be passed into the ureter without a guidewire, thus minimizing the role of the semi-rigid ureteroscope [4, 5]. With improvement in distal active tip deflection, having a larger diameter with a maximum angle of the deflection of 270°, the endoscope could be passed through the intra-mural ureter under direct vision, and then proximally into the kidney [5]. A semirigid instrument was no longer required for all cases, employing a flexible instrument solely. Thus, as the fiberoptic endoscopes were miniaturized, the ability to evaluate an upper tract urothelial lesion in a particularly atraumatic fashion expanded (Fig. 4.1b). Complications decreased significantly, while the ability of the surgeon to map the collecting system broadened.

The strategy employed in evaluating an upper urinary tract filling defect or a suspicious lesion defined on contrast enhanced CT/MRI that is felt to be urothelial in origin, is based on first performing a careful diagnostic cystoscopy. Bladder barbotage urine specimens for cytopathology are obtained. Retrograde ureteropyelography is then performed with dilute contrast medium, helping to define areas that are particularly suspicious (Fig. 4.2). The flexible ureteroscope is then passed into the ureteral orifice under direct vision, if technically feasible. If the endoscope does not pass easily through the intramural tunnel, then a guidewire is placed through the instrument intubating the orifice as an obturator. If the endoscope continues to fail to pass thru the intramural segment, then a dilator is employed. Either a balloon or graduated dilator, no more than 12 French in diameter, is then employed to minimally dilate the intramural segment and thus decrease false positive findings on direct endoscopy.

When mapping the upper urinary tract urothelium, the flexible endoscope is passed up the

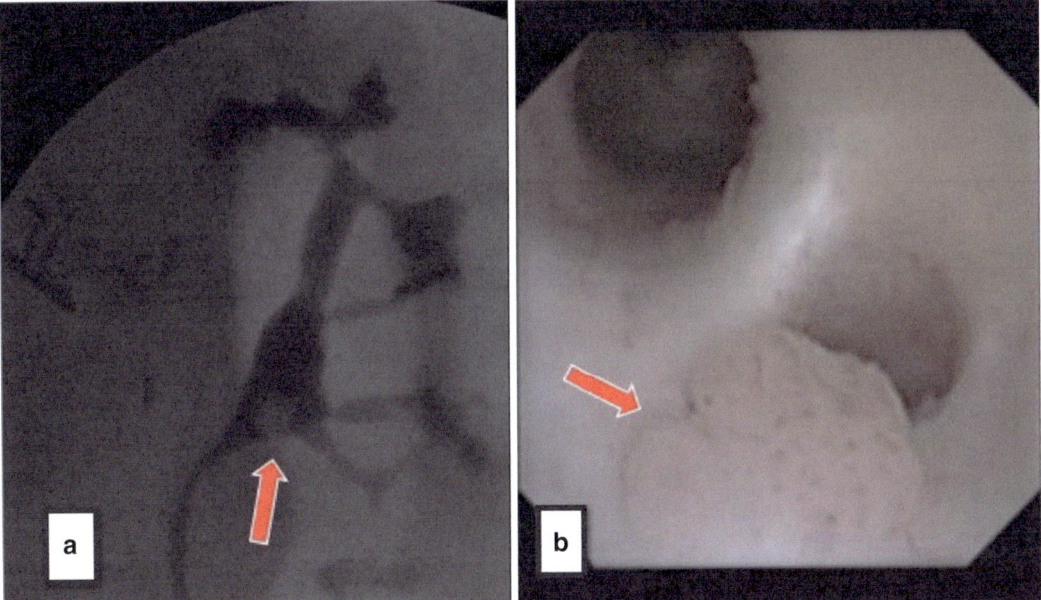

Fig. 4.2 (a) Left retrograde pyelogram depicting clear circular filling defect in renal pelvis (*red arrow*). (b) The digital flexible ureteroscope gives clear visual confirmation of tumor (*red arrow*) corresponding to filling defect

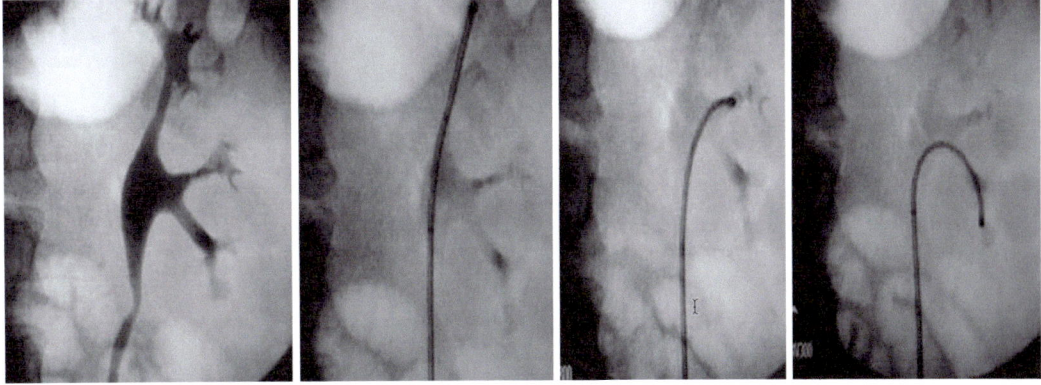

Fig. 4.3 The actively deflectable flexible ureteroscope allows for meticulous inspection/mapping of the entire intrarenal collecting system, thereby serving as the primary tool for diagnosis and treatment of upper tract pathology

ureter under direct vision using sterile saline irrigant to clear the operative field. A barbotage specimen of saline is collected through the working channel of the endoscope during this evaluation for cytopathology. The intrarenal collecting system is carefully and meticulously inspected (Fig. 4.3). Suspicious lesions are sampled. For a papillary lesion (Fig. 4.5a), the application of a 2.4 French stainless steel based flat wire basket is an excellent accessory to obtain adequate tissue for histopathology. Tissue from the lesion is engaged in the basket, and a portion removed by extracting the endoscope and basket as a unit (Fig. 4.4). Specifically the basket is not pulled back through the working channel, rather the engaged tissue basket and endoscope are removed as a unit such that a sizable portion of tumor can be sent for histopathology. The endoscope is then replaced, and if the resultant hematuria associated with the biopsy is minimal, then additional

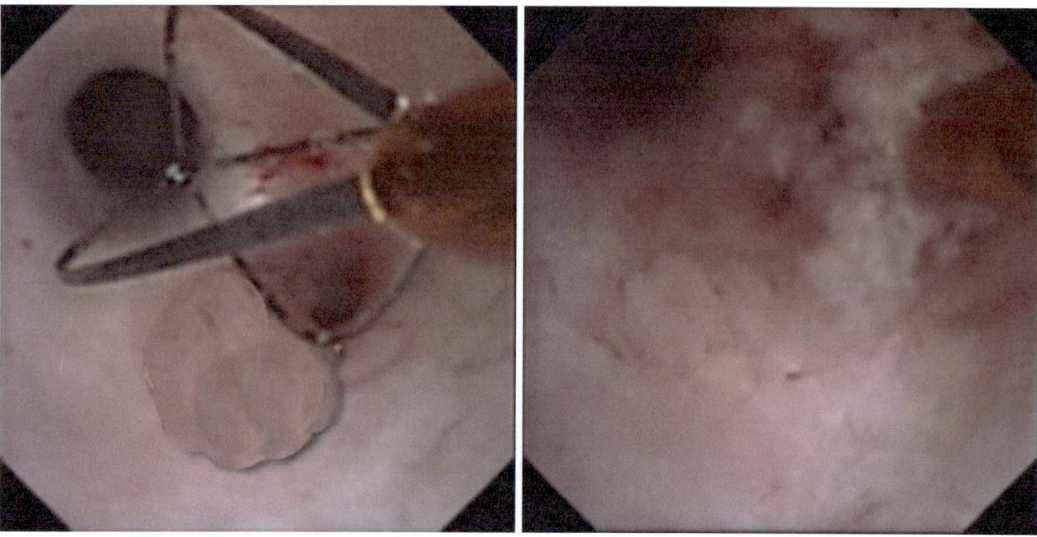

Fig. 4.4 2.4 Fr Segura stainless steel basket is used to ensnare the tumor and obtain tissue for biopsy and pathological diagnosis

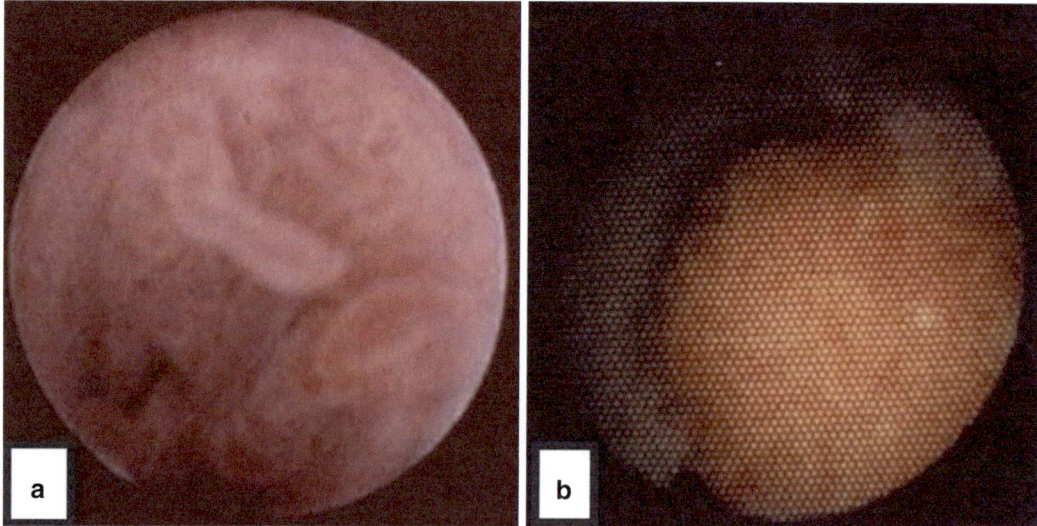

Fig. 4.5 (**a**) Endoscopic appearance of a papillary, low grade lesion- note shaggy appearance of frons with fibrovascular cores. (**b**) A high grade lesion, on the other hand, tends to be flat (sessile) and broad based

biopsies and a second barbotage specimen for cytopathology is collected.

Flat, sessile, or small papillary lesions are difficult to biopsy ureteroscopically with a snare or flat wire basket (Fig. 4.5b). In those settings a small cup biopsy forceps is employed. The specimen, which is often a millimeter or smaller in size, is collected by extracting the forceps through the endoscope's working channel. Multiple samplings with the cup forceps increase the sensitivity of this technique. The tiny specimens are released from the forceps by plunging the open cups into a conical tube under a few cc's of saline. Multiple pieces are obtained of a suspicious flat area for example, with the specimen then prepared by the cytopathologist [6]. The conical tube is spun down to obtain a small tissue pellet, which is prepared employing cell block technique to improve the sensitivity of the biopsy. The supernatant is evaluated cytologically as well [6–8]. After ureteroscopic biopsy, another barbotage specimen is collected thru the endoscope's working channel to help define any high-grade cells that may have been released with the act of mechanical biopsy, improving the sensitivity of the diagnostic procedure.

Commonly after performing an ureteroscopic biopsy, an internal ureteral stent will be placed to better ensure that the upper urinary tract remains drained. Frequently after a biopsy there will be associated hematuria. By employing a small electrocautery probe or laser energy through the ureteroscope, the base of the biopsy site can be coagulated for hemostasis, but frequently after the biopsy the involved segment is coated with a small portion of clot prohibiting this manuever. It is in that setting that a ureteral catheter is placed to help ensure drainage, minimizing clot colic, after this diagnostic procedure. Please see Chapter 1 for further discussion of diagnostic ureteroscopy.

4.3   Therapeutic Ureteropyeloscopy for Upper Urinary Tract Urothelial Malignancies: Technical Considerations

The treatment of upper urinary tract urothelial lesions varies based on the grade, structure, size, vascularity, and location of the encountered tumor [9]. Grade on presentation is the most significant prognosticator, and should direct to a large extent the crafted treatment algorithm [10–12]. Here again we mirror the experience in the lower urinary tract, where low grade lesions are often definitively treated, but recurrences are common and progression in grade with a recurrence will radically change therapy. Patients treated ureteroscopically in this setting must by counseled from the onset of therapy that lifelong endoscopic surveillance is an essential part of treatment. In addition post treatment surveillance

includes periodic urine and serum studies, as well as additional imaging to define progression in stage [13].

Ureteroscopic therapy often begins with tissue sampling for histopathology, cytologic washings, and additional imaging studies for staging including standard imaging to assess for metastatic disease. After these baseline studies are completed, they are repeated at an interval over time to define recurrence and/or progression in grade and stage. Ureteroscopic treatment is employed in various settings: as definitive therapy in those with low grade lesions and favorable cytology, to palliate a symptomatic high grade lesion (e.g. addressing hematuria, un-obstructing the collecting system, etc.), or in those patients with high grade lesions who are not candidates for extirpative surgery secondary to co-morbidities or who refuse nephroureterectomy which may leave them with marginal renal function understanding that this therapy is most often palliative in this setting.

In the past, the majority of distal ureteral tumors were endoscopically treated with a 12 French uretero-resectoscope (Fig. 4.6). The addition and universal acceptance of small diameter fiberoptic semirigid endoscopes and actively deflectable, flexible ureteroscopes has led to abandonment of the larger and more traumatic instruments, rendering them almost obsolete. Current use of the uretero-resectoscope is, therefore, very limited and generally reserved for the largest distal ureteral tumors in a particularly dilated collecting system [14].

Papillary tumors that have bland papillae (Figs. 4.5a and 4.7) which are not particularly vascular can be treated with either electrocautery or holmium:YAG laser energy [15, 16]. The energy setting with regard to holmium laser energy is lower than those employed for lithotripsy. Low laser energies of 0.4–0.6 J, and frequency of pulsation that varies between 5 and 10 Hz, are common settings. Lower settings will ablate tumor while also coagulating the lesion, minimizing hematuria while maintaining a clear optical field (Fig. 4.8). Lesions that are papillary with sizable vascular cores and/or are particularly friable tend to bleed even with minimal manipulation and require a different treatment strategy.

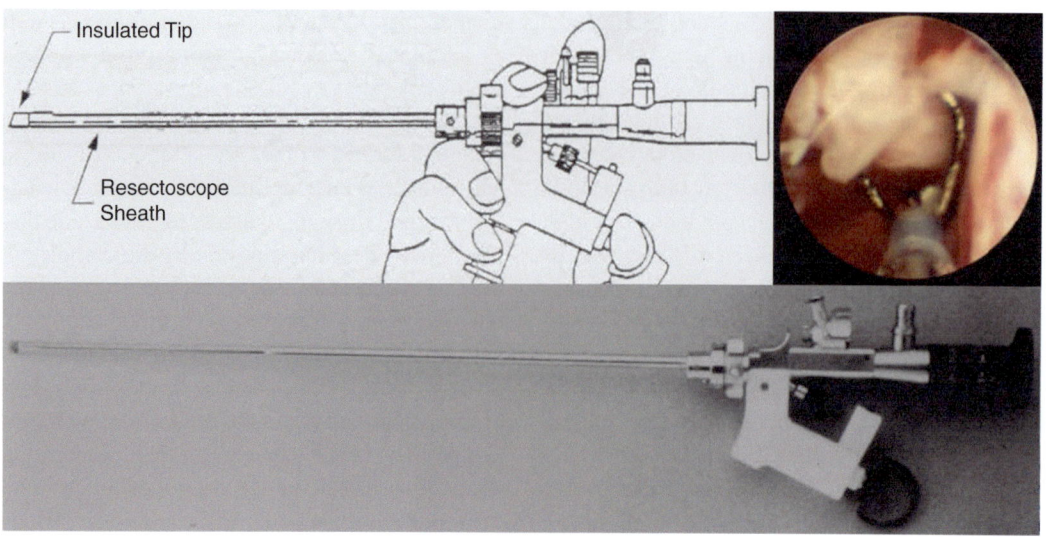

Fig. 4.6 The uretero-resectoscope being used to resect a distal ureteral papillary tumor (*inset*)

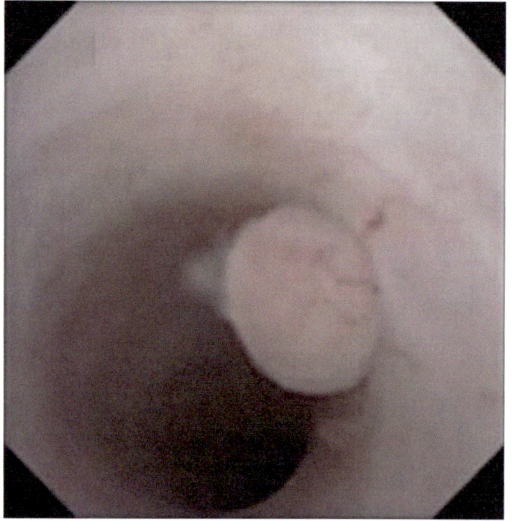

Fig. 4.7 Ureteroscopic view of a superficial, low grade urothelial tumor in the mid ureter

In that setting the base of the lesion is initially either coagulated with a 2 French Bugbee electrode or Nd:YAG laser energy is employed to de-vascularize the stalk, with subsequent application of holmium laser energy to remove (i.e. resect) the frons. The Nd:YAG laser settings are lower than what is employed for other solid tissue applications. Twenty to 30 W of power, employed for short periods though-out the visible tumor,

will give optimal coagulation of the lesion, with holmium laser energy subsequently employed to clear (i.e. resect or ablate) the de-vascularized frons. It is important to note that higher settings of Nd:YAG laser energy applied for longer periods of time can be associated with significant tissue fibrosis, and can also create a sizeable acute soft tissue defect that can be associated with bleeding [17]. To minimize this, Nd:YAG laser wavelength should be used with lower power employed to a site for shorter periods. In addition, this wavelength should be used sparingly in the ureter, never circumferentially which has been associated with a high stricture rate.

Ureteroscopic treatment can obtain local control for particularly vascular high grade lesions but in general this treatment is commonly palliative [9, 10]. The most common presenting symptom is significant gross hematuria, where the surgeon is asked to stop the bleeding endoscopically. In that setting both Nd:YAG laser energy and electrocautery can be employed successfully. For lesions within the intra-renal collecting system, Nd:YAG laser energy can be employed around the tumor initially, from peripheral to central, in a non-contact mode, defocusing the light energy to create an area of thermal coagulation. Nd:Yag is avidly absorbed by hemoglobin, thus vascular lesions absorb this

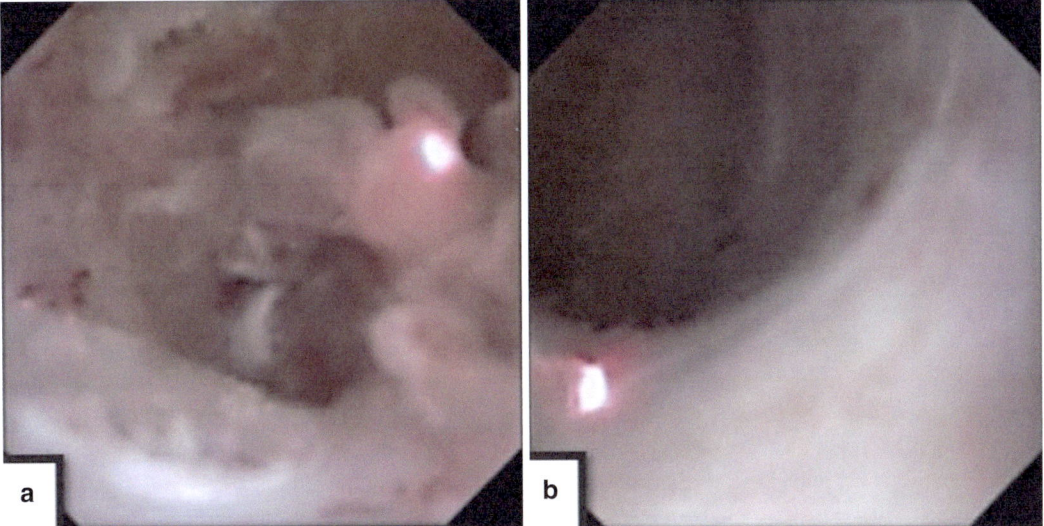

Fig. 4.8 Large volume papillary tumor filing a calyx (**a**) is carefully treated here with holmium:YAG laser energy resulting in clearance of tumor burden, down to flat mucosa (**b**)

wavelength readily facilitating a deep coagulative effect [18, 19]. Electrocautery commonly produces a crust of coagulated tissue which may inhibit the efficiency of laser energy applied on the same tissue thereafter. In this setting of significant hematuria small aliquots of sterile water, limited to a small finite volume (i.e. less than 200 cc's), will often clear the optical filed sufficiently so an energy source can be employed precisely to stop bleeding. It also important to remember that complete treatment commonly requires staged therapy, where coagulated tumor is allowed to slough, exposing the residua at the second sitting. Alternatively, holmium:YAG can be employed intermittently after Nd:Yag therapy to actively remove coagulated tumor exposing the lesions' base.

Low grade lesions, specifically tumors that are biopsy proven low grade on histopathology and free of high grade cells on cytopathology from washings, are commonly treated ureteroscopically with the intent to cure [11–13]. Lesions that are large, either within in the intrarenal collecting system or ureter, and those that are circumferential in the ureter are often treated in stages. Treating a section of the ureteral wall, for example, and then allowing a period of healing with re-epithelialization before completing

treatment minimizes the risk of stricture associated with thermal energy applied in this way. With ureteroscopic treatment of an extensive tumor burden, tumor is ablated at the first sitting, a ureteral stent is placed, and then patient returns after a short interval of healing (i.e. 1–2 weeks) for additional treatment after the devitalized tissue is allowed to slough. Staged therapy is also employed when extensive and/or multifocal tumor resection is required and when visualization is compromised due to bleeding during primary endoscopic resection [14].

For sizable intrarenal lesions that are particularly vascular, Nd:YAG laser energy can be employed to de-vascularize the lesion, with holmium laser energy employed immediately thereafter as a resecting wavelength. Applying these two laser wavelengths in sequence can efficiently remove a sizeable low grade lesion. A ureteral stent is regularly placed after the initial treatment, maintaining drainage while tumor sloughs, edema from thermal therapy resolves, especially between staged resections. Employing the staged methodology can facilitate clearance of even sizable lesions. Other relative indications for ureteral stenting post ureteroscopic treatment include a solitary renal unit, tumor multifocality, and tumor that is located in the intra-mural ureter.

A period of stenting will better ensure drainage, and also during this period of healing, will allow the urothelium to regenerate in areas that were treated with one of the energy sources employed.

The endoscopist must be keenly aware of the limitations of the energy sources employed. Laser energy delivered in a pulsatile fashion will clear tumor similar to resection in the bladder, developing a smooth surface without visible tumor at the end of the treatment. Limits of laser energy though include the relatively stiff laser fibers that can inhibit the flexibility of the endoscope. Smaller diameter laser fibers are employed for lesions in the peripheral intrarenal collecting system, specifically in the lower pole. Lesions that are located in a peripheral calyx can be challenging to treat, particularly if tumor resides under the lip of a calyx or in a tortuous infundibulum. The holmium:YAG laser used at low energy can effectively coagulate tumor when placed in close proximity to a papillary projection. However, if a laser fiber cannot be focused directly on the tumor, i.e. under a calyceal lip to treat a rim of residual tumor, then a small 2 French electrocautery probe is often successful. The electrical energy is delivered circumferentially, as opposed to linearly from the tip of the laser fiber. The 2 French electrode can thus be placed adjacent to a tumor, and using either cutting or coagulation current the lesion is treated adjacent to the tip of the probe.

4.4 The Application of Adjuvant Topical Agents to Maximize Ureteroscopic Treatment of Upper Urinary Tract Urothelial Tumors

Various agents can be employed topically in the upper urinary tract to maximize therapy and minimize recurrence of an upper tract urothelial tumor, similar to their application in the lower urinary tract. Commonly this is employed immediately after ureteroscopic treatment, mirroring applications in the bladder immediately after transurethral resection [20]. Mitomycin C is the most frequently employed topical agent applied in the upper urinary tract [21–24].

From a technical perspective, the application of topical chemotherapeutic agents in the upper urinary tract requires an externally draining catheter. A single pigtail stent of relatively small diameter, most commonly 6 French, is employed which is secured to a bladder drainage (i.e. foley) catheter during treatment. This ureteral stent is positioned post ureteroscopic treatment into the upper urinary tract with the proximal pigtail precisely coiled in a predetermined segment of the intrarenal collecting system, preventing inadvertent instillation into tissue. In contrast, if an open ended catheter is employed the tip may inadvertently contact tissue, increasing the risk of absorption with significant systemic risk. For this reason as a routine the pigtail catheter's position should be verified with contrast fluoroscopically before instillation of the topical agent.

A small aliquot of contrast (e.g. 2–10 cc's depending on the volume of the intrarenal collecting system) is employed through the catheter with simultaneous real time fluoroscopic imaging to obtain a retrograde ureteropyelogram. If significant extravasation is noted at the end of the ureteroscopic procedure during this maneuver, then the application of the topical chemotherapy should be delayed and the catheter set to gravity until the upper urinary tract seals.

Mitomycin C solution for upper tract instillation most commonly is 20 mg in 100 cc of diluent. This is administered in a retrograde fashion through a single pigtail catheter over the course of approximately 1 h. Administration is carried out in the recovery room immediately after endoscopic treatment. This is a setting where patients can be carefully and continuously monitored during the treatment. The nursing staff is keenly aware of parameters that lead to stoppage of the instillation: specifically flank pain, fever, nausea and emesis, which all may reflect increased intrarenal pressure. Mitomycin solution is never actively pumped into the upper tract, but rather administered by gravity drip. If the intrarenal pressures are high reflecting obstruction then the gravity drip will stop, thus minimizing the risk of systemic absorption. Mitimycin C is also a topical irritant and can cause severe skin reactions. Patients are padded under their buttock and genitalia to collect any leakage from incontinence around the catheters. The mito-mycin solution has a purple dye marker, and the nursing staff is clear that if they encounter this on the padding that the patient is immediately cleansed to minimize contact dermatitis and skin reaction.

The application of topical chemotherapy in the upper urinary tract is infrequently employed at the time of initial diagnostic ureteroscopy, and is most frequently employed in those patients with recurrence following a surveillance protocol after definitive therapy, or as part of staged ure-teroscopic treatment for a sizeable or complex lesion. During surveillance, indications for topi-cal therapy include either a sizeable or multifocal recurrence, or if the interval between recurrences is shortening. In those settings topical therapy is employed to minimize recurrence. Patients are carefully counseled on the risks associated with topical therapy, very similar to the counseling when this agent is employed in the bladder. See chapter X for further discussion of topical therapy.

4.5   Antegrade Endoscopic Treatment of Upper Urinary Tract Urothelial Malignancies

Before advanced retrograde flexible ureteropy-eloscopic instrumentation became available, antegrade percutaneous endoscopic techniques were employed to treat upper urinary tract uro-thelial malignancies. The tenets of this form of endoscopic treatment were a staged placement of percutaneous access into the kidney, commonly allowing the tract to mature, followed by rigid endoscopic technique to treat papillary urothelial tumors. Limitations included the rigid instru-ments that were being employed which often could not access the entire intrarenal collecting system, the relatively high rate of significant hematuria requiring transfusion perioperatively, and the risk of tract seeding [25]. The addition of the flexible nephroscope, and subsequently the actively deflectable flexible ureteropyeloscope placed in an antegrade fashion down the ureter,

broadened the indications for treatment and improved success rates in general [26].

Published series of patients with intrarenal urothelial malignancies treated in a percutaneous antegrade fashion have had relatively short fol-low-up with, in general, acceptable perioperative outcomes [27, 28]. The risk profile, however, associated with antegrade endoscopic treatment of an intrarenal urothelial tumor when compared to retrograde technique is significantly higher. Not only is there a higher risk of significant hematuria associated with this antegrade endo-scopic resection, but the risk increases exponen-tially with repetitive procedures. Moreover, endoscopic surveillance protocols would logi-cally be carried out using retrograde uretero-scopic technique henceforth. Thus the indications for antegrade endoscopic treatment of intrarenal urothelial malignancies are limited to those patients where retrograde access is not techni-cally feasible (e.g. those with urinary diversions or a lower urinary tract reconstruction that prohibits retrograde access) or patients who for technical reasons the standard retrograde ure-teropyeloscopic techniques are ineffective. One example is a patient with a large bulky papillary tumor where antegrade technique would more efficiently clear this significant volume of malig-nant tissue as compared to retrograde instrumen-tation requiring multiple sessions. Once again, this has to be weighed against the significantly higher risk of bleeding and potential renal loss from a percutaneous access in this setting. On the opposite side of the efficiency argument is the fact that relatively large lesions have been treated successfully ureteroscopically with significantly less morbidity [25, 29]. Retrograde treatment may require staged interventions to allow treated tumor to slough between applications of one of a variety of energy sources employed to coagulate visible tumor.

In summary, antegrade endoscopic treatment of an upper urinary tract urothelial malignancy has a limited role. The complications associated with this procedure are significantly greater than those associated with retrograde ureteroscopic therapy. The role of employing antegrade percu-taneous tumor therapy is relegated to a select population of patients where retrograde access is not technically feasible, or in those patients where retrograde technique would be impractical based on clinical parameters defined at the time of presentation.

4.6 Retrograde Ureteropyeloscopic Treatment of Upper Urinary Tract Urothelial Malignancies Compared to Nephroureterectomy: Initial Success and Long-Term Outcomes

The published literature with regard to ureteroscopic treatment of upper urinary tract urothelial malignancies is limited, due to the relatively low incidence of this disease as compared to lower urinary tract tumors, the varied treatment protocols that were employed at various tertiary referral centers, and issues with regard to careful surveillance of the patient population defining long-term outcomes. We have carefully and fastidiously followed a patient population over 15 years with upper urinary tract urothelial lesions treated both ureteroscopically and with nephroureterectomy. This data has been published in sequence at different points of maturity, with the most recent 15-year follow-up presented in the British Journal of Urology in 2013 [29]. The presented database reflects a population of patients presenting with upper urinary tract urothelial tumors who were differentiated initially by grade at the time of diagnostic ureteroscopy and then placed in one of three treatment groups (Table 4.1).

Patients with low-grade urothelial tumors, irrespective of size and location, who either had comorbidities that prohibited nephroureterectomy or who had the potential risk of progressing to end-stage renal disease with nephroureterectomy were offered ureteroscopic treatment with concurrent lifelong ureteroscopic surveillance ("Group 1"- see Table 4.1). In this group, all patients agreed at the onset of treatment to be followed with at minimum annual

ureteroscopic surveillance from the onset of the treatment protocol. The definition of a low-grade upper tract urothelial tumor was comprised of two data points, one being a biopsy of the lesions in question that reflected a low-grade histopathology, and also cytologic review of barbotage washings of the upper urinary tract that defined no high-grade cells, thus minimizing any risk of a concurrent high-grade lesions or carcinoma in situ. With this as the starting point, the patients underwent either complete or staged ureteroscopic resection to render them tumor free, with subsequent sequential surveillance ureteroscopies initially on a quarterly basis, but ultimately with negative evaluations on an annual basis. In addition, annual CT or MR imaging as part of a metastatic evaluation was performed, with semiannual cystoscopic bladder inspections and cytopathologic review of either voided urine or barbotage specimen at the time of cystoscopy.

A second smaller group of patients who presented with symptomatic high-grade upper tract urothelial lesions who either refused nephroureterectomy, could not tolerate nephroureterectomy based on comorbidities, or would not tolerate lifelong hemodialysis if nephroureterectomy was employed were offered palliative ureteroscopic treatment ("Group 2"- see Table 4.1). All patients in this group from the onset of treatment understood that they had a particularly high risk of progression to metastatic disease, and that ureteroscopic treatment was being employed solely in a palliative fashion to minimize or obviate the clinical symptoms that led to their presentation. These symptoms included significant gross hematuria, upper urinary tract obstruction, etc.

The last group of patients in the study reflects all patients who after initial diagnosis were treated with nephroureterectomy ("Group 3"- see Table 4.1). The majority of these patients underwent a laparoscopic nephroureterectomy. All patients underwent regional lymph node sampling as part of staging. This group of patients had a higher proportion of high-grade tumors as compared to other series, based in part on the fact that ureteroscopic intervention for the low-grade

Table 4.1 Patient demographics and findings at initial diagnosis

| | URS groups | | Extirpative surgery group | |
	Group 1	Group 2	Group 3	All groups
No. of patients	66	14	80	**160**
Median age (range)	73 (45–93)	71.5 (48–89)	72.5 (46–90)	**73 (45–93)**
Sex. n (%)				
Male	35 (53)	11	50 (62.5)	**96 (60)**
Female	31 (47)	3	30 (37.5)	**64 (40)**
Mean age-adjusted CCI (range)	5.5 (0–13)	7.1 (2–11)	5.1 (0–13)	**5.4 (0–13)**
Initial/last follow-up mean creatinine concentration, mg/dL	1.5/1.7	2.0/2.5	13/1.6	**1.4/1.7**
Solitary kidney, n (%)	17 (25.8)	6	2 (2.5)	**25 (15.6)**
Bilateral disease, n (%)	9 (13.6)	5	4 (5)	**18 (11.3)**
Multifocality, n (%)	21 (31.8%)	11	23 (28.8)	**55 (34.4)**
Urothelial cancer, n (%)				
Preoperative history of bladder cancer	29 (43.9)	10	21 (26.3)	**60 (37.5)**
High grade	9 (13.6)	7	12 (15)	**28 (17.5)**
Low grade	23 (34.8)	4	11 (13.8)	**38 (23.8)**
Concomitant bladder cancer	17 (25.8)	5	20 (25)	**42 (26.3)**
History of cystectomy	1 (1.5)	4	1 (1.3)	**6 (3.0)**
Preoperative history of upper tract cancer	19 (28.8)	7	6 (7.5)	**32 (20)**
High grade	6 (9.1)	3	0 (0)	**9 (5.6)**
Low grade	13 (19.7)	4	6 (7.5)	**23 (14.4)**
Initial grade at diagnosis, n (%)				
High grade	0 (0)	14	57 (71.3)	**71 (44.4)**
Low grade	66 (100)	0	23 (28.8)	**89 (55.6)**
Initial upper tract tumour, n (%)				
Large: >3 cm	18 (27.3)	9	62 (77.5)	**89 (55.6)**
Medium: 1–3 cm	32 (48.5)	2	14 (17.5)	**48 (30)**
Small: <1 cm	16 (24.2)	3	4 (5)	**23 (14.4)**
Mean size, cm	2.3	3.07	3.5	**3.0**
Mean (range) follow-up, months	51.5 (3–166.4)	25.1 (6.5–47.8)	30.4 (1–185.3)	**38.2 (1–185.3)**

Group 1 low grade upper tract tumors managed ureteroscopically (ureteroscopic therapy group), *Group 2* high grade upper tract tumors managed ureteroscopically (palliative group), *Group 3* upper tract tumors managed with nephroureterectomy (extirpative therapy group) [29]

lesions was offered as treatment as well, and so many of those patients were obviously treated in that fashion and not with removal of the upper urinary tract. Those treated with nephroureterectomy were also carefully followed with serial cystoscopic evaluations of the bladder with cytologies, and frequent metastatic evaluations with either CT or MR imaging.

The patients who presented with low-grade disease and were treated ureteroscopically (Group 1) had very similar long-term cancer specific survival as compared to those treated with nephroureterectomy (Fig. 4.9). As we note commonly in the bladder, small low grade recurrences in other portions of the collecting system were frequent (Fig. 4.10) [30]. Of those patients with low-grade disease treated ureteroscopically, the progression in grade was found to be 15.2 % to high grade, with a mean time of 38.5 months (Table 4.2). In those that progressed in grade, many progressed in stage, underscoring the importance of lifelong ureteroscopic surveillance. Thus, ureteroscopic

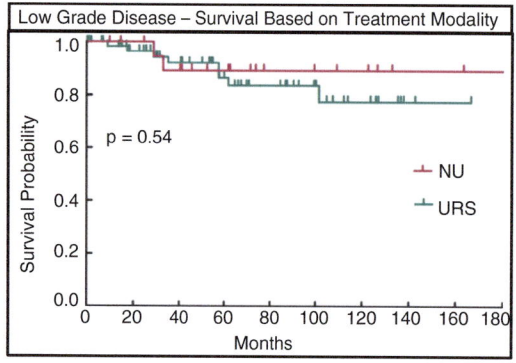

Fig. 4.9 Cancer-specific survival (CSS) of all patients with **low grade disease** stratified by treatment method. *NU* nephroureterectomy, *URS* ureteroscopically treated group (Group 1) [29]

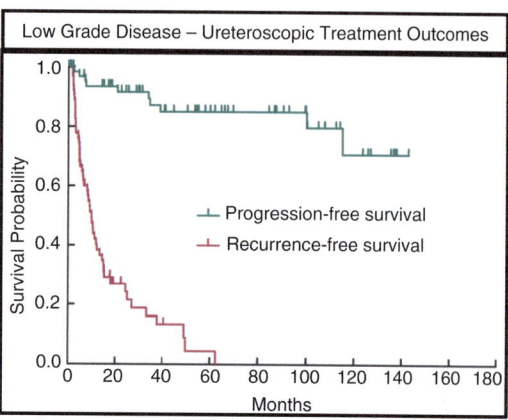

Fig. 4.10 Recurrence- and progression-free survival of patients with <u>**low grade disease**</u> treated with ureteroscopy (Group 1). Note frequent recurrences that mimic natural history of urothelial cancer as seen in the bladder [29]

Table 4.2 Perioperative data and outcomes of ureteroscopic management

	Group 1 (Low Grade)	*Group 2 (High Grade)*
Number of Patients	66	14
Total Number of URS	522	75
Mean number of URS per patient	7.9	5.4
Staged URS Required for Tumor Clearance	14.9%	38%
Urothelial Recurrence		
Upper Tract Recurrence	51 (77.3%)	14 (100%)
Median Time to 1st Recurrence (Months) (Range)	9.9 (1.1-62.3)	3 (1-8)
New Bladder Cancer	18 (27.2%)	2 (14.3%)
Bladder Recurrence	40 (60.6%)	7 (50%)
Progression		
Progression to High Grade	10 (15.2%)	NA
Undergraded Initial URS Biopsy (Subsequent Biopsy in < 6 months High Grade)	3 (4.5%)	NA
Overgraded on Survelliance URS Bioopsy	2 (3%)	NA
Subsequent Nephroureterectomy	11 (16.7%)	4 (28.6%)
Progression to Renal Failure	4 (6.1%)	5 (35.7%)
Survival Analysis		
Deceased	20 (30.3%)	12 (85.7%)
Median Overall Survival (Months)	126.8	29.2
Cancer Related Deaths	8 (12.1%)	12 (85.7%)
Metastasis	9 (13.6.%)	13 (92.9%)

Red box denotes a finding of 15 % progression to high grade in our ureteroscopic therapy group (Group 1) [29]

treatment with careful, meticulous surveillance was felt to have an acceptable oncologic endpoint, and thus reflects a standard therapy for patients presenting with these parameters. The 2, 5, and 10-year cancer specific survival rates in this low grade group were 97, 87, and 78 %, very similar to those patients with low grade disease treated with nephroureterectomy (Table 4.3).

As a stark contrast to patients with low-grade disease treated ureteroscopically, those with high-grade disease treated with nephroureterectomy were often not cured with extirpative treatment (Fig. 4.11). The 2, 5, and 10-year cancer free survival were 70, 53, and 38 %, with a metastatic free survival of 55, 45, and 35 %. When this data is compared to a series of nephroureterectomies performed at the Cleveland Clinic, cancer specific survival was notably comparable

at long term follow-up [31]. The difference in the two patient populations reflects a higher proportion of patients in the New York series with high-grade disease, and the fact that there was a higher incidence of positive regional lymph nodes. This can be explained from a technical perspective in that routinely a wide lymph node dissection looking for metastatic disease was performed, where as at other centers this is not necessarily a routine. Beyond grade, survival following nephroureterectomy was influenced significantly by final pathologic stage of the tumor and the presence of lymph node metastases (Fig. 4.12).

The overall and cancer-specific survival in all three treatment groups is presented in Table 4.3 and Fig. 4.13. The group of patients with high-grade disease treated ureteroscopically

Table 4.3 Overall, cancer specific and metastasis-free survival outcomes [29]

	2 year (%)			5 year (%)			10 year (%)		
	Overall	Cancer specific	Metastasis-free	Overall	Cancer specific	Metastasis-free	Overall	Cancer specific	Metastasis-free
All groups (n = 160)	82	84	76	59	67	64	40	59	58
Initial grade at URS presentation									
Low	95	98	95	76	87	85	59	81	81
High	64	65	50	33	35	33	0	23	23
Ureteroscopic management									
Group 1 (LG – treatment)	93	97	97	74	87	84	56	78	75
Group 2 (HG – palliative)	54	54	34	0	0	0	0	0	0
Extirpative surgery									
Group 3 (NU)	77	78	66	58	64	60	36	56	54
Pathologic stage									
Ta-Tis-TI	91	94	86	78	86	78	52	80	74
Low grade	100	100	95	88	93	95	73	93	95
High grade	83	88	78	68	78	61	€	58	51
T2	91	91	74	54	67	65	54	67	65
T3	49	49	32	22	22	0	0	0	0
T4	25	25	0	25	25	0	25	25	0
Lymph node positive	24	24	NA	0	0	NA	0	0	NA
Pathologic grade on NU									
Low	100	100	91	79	89	91	66	89	91
High	67	70	55	47	53	45	0	38	35

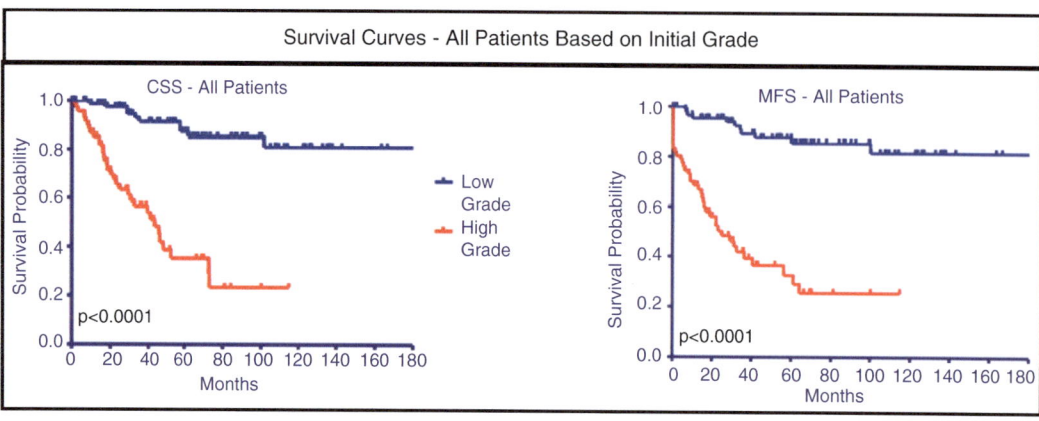

Fig. 4.11 Cancer- Specific (*CSS*) and Metastatic-Free (*MFS*) Survival of all patients based on initial grade of tumor [29]

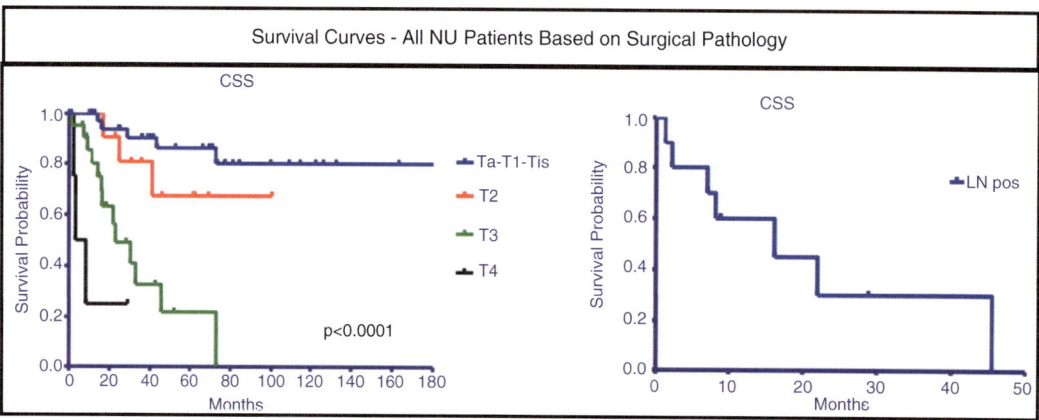

Fig. 4.12 Cancer- Specific Survival (*CSS*) of all patients who underwent nephroureterectomy (*NU*) stratified by stage and lymph node positivity [29]

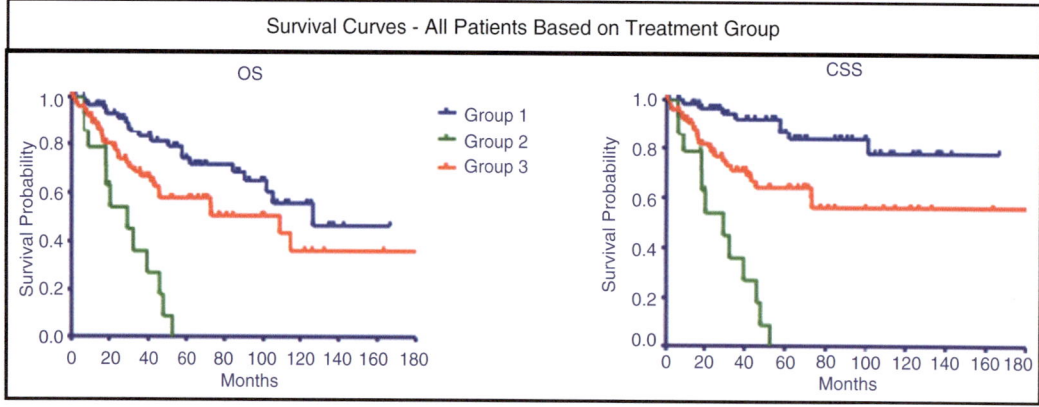

Fig. 4.13 Overall (*OS*) and Cancer-Specific (*CSS*) Survival of all patients treated for upper tract urothelial carcinoma. (*Group 1* ureteroscopic therapy group, *Group 2* palliative group, *Group 3* extirpative therapy group) [29]

(i.e. Group 2) all progressed in stage, and all succumbed to the disease. The median survival of patients in this group with high grade lesions treated ureteroscopically was 29.2 months, with a 2-year survival rate of 54 %. Placing this in context, all patients in this group presented with serious acute and/or life ending symptoms where ureteroscopic intervention improved quality and quantity of life, but was not curative. The median survival in this group treated in this fashion was higher than in other series where ureteroscopy was employed [32, 33]. This may reflect the application of staged therapies to address complex intrarenal and ureteral lesions, with the intent to obviate acute symptoms (e.g. gross hematuria, severe colic, complete obstruction) and improve upper urinary tract drainage.

What is clear from this data is that tumor grade is by far the most significant predictor of overall and cancer-specific survival in those patients presenting with upper tract malignancies regardless of surgical intervention (Table 4.4). Both ureteroscopic and extirpative interventions

for low-grade lesions has merit and should be employed routinely in those patients with low-grade disease. Where nephroureterectomy would leave them with minimal residual renal function, ureteroscopic intervention should be employed with the caveat that lifelong ureteroscopic surveillance is required. Those patients should be counseled that there is a 15 % risk of progression in grade on surveillance, not unlike what is defined with lower urinary tract malignancies, and thus meticulous follow-up including lifelong ureteroscopic surveillance is mandatory.

These oncologic outcomes are similar to what Tolley et al published in 2012 [9]. Although this Scottish 20 year experience did not stratify patients according to tumor grade, the CSS at 5 and 10 years were similar at 88.9 and 77.4 %. A comparable rate of disease progression was identified at 19.2 %.

In those patients with high-grade disease treated with nephroureterectomy, the data on overall cancer-specific survival is sobering. It is clear that nephroureterectomy alone often does

Table 4.4 Predictive variables of overall and cancer specific survival using univariate and multivariate analysis

	Overall Survival						Cancer Specific Survival					
	Univariate Analysis			Multivariate Analysis			Univariate Analysis			Multivariate Analysis		
Prognostic Variables	HR	95% CI	p Value	HR	95% CI	p Value	HR	95% CI	p Value	HR	95% CI	p Value
Age (≥ 73)	1.48	(0.90 - 2.45)	0.126				1.19	(0.66 - 2.14)	0.571			
Sex (M/F)	1.31	(0.79 - 2.17)	0.314				1.57	(0.87 - 2.86)	0.157			
Age Adjusted CCI (≥ 6)	2.28	(1.36 - 3.82)	0.002*	2.01	(1.16 - 3.46)	0.012*	2.03	(1.11 - 3.71)	0.021*	1.88	(0.98 - 3.6)	0.056
Preop Bladder Cancer (Y/N)	1.87	(1.09 - 3.22)	0.627	1.39	(0.78 - 2.47)	0.27	1.87	(1.00 - 3.51)	0.034*	1.10	(0.55 - 2.18)	
Concomitant Bladder Tumor (Y/N)	0.79	(0.44 - 1.42)	0.46				0.68	(0.34 - 1.34)	0.313			
Initial Upper Tract Tumor Grade (High/Low)	3.76	(2.16 - 6.53)	<.0001*	3.78	(2.11 - 6.80)	<.0001*	7.27	(3.86 - 13.71)	<.0001*	7.14	(3.25 - 15.7)	<.0001*
Initial Tumor Size (>3cm)	1.56	(0.95 - 2.59)	0.082				2.29	(1.27 - 4.13)	0.008*	1.74	(0.88 - 3.44)	0.11
Bilateral Disease (Y/N)	1.09	(0.51 - 2.35)	0.82				1.43	(0.57 - 3.59)	0.382			
Solitary Kidney (Y/N)	0.86	(0.44 - 1.68)	0.67				0.95	(0.43 - 2.09)	0.892			
Multifocality (Y/N)	1.25	(0.74 - 2.13)	0.39				1.76	(0.94 - 3.28)	0.058	1.28	(0.65 - 2.50)	0.47
Bladder Recurrence (Y/N)	0.58	(0.35 - 0.96)	0.031*	0.65	(0.38 - 1.12)	0.12	0.60	(0.33 - 1.09)	0.089			
Progression to Renal Failure (Y/N)	2.94	(1.04 - 8.27)	0.001*	1.44	(0.83 - 3.79)	0.14	4.04	(1.25 - 13.06)	<.0001*	2.28	(0.96 - 5.45)	0.06

* Significant at p <.05 (Statistically significant values on univariate analysis were selected for multivariate analysis)

Red box denotes overwhelming significance of grade on survival outcome
CCI Charlson Comorbidity Index [29]

not lead to a long-term cancer-specific survival. As with urothelial tumors of the lower urinary tract, both adjuvant and neoadjuvant systemic chemotherapeutic regimens can be employed in an attempt to improve long-term survival. A recent meta-analysis questioned the routine use of systemic chemotherapy in this setting [34]. What is clear from this grouping of retrospective reviews is that cisplatinum based chemotherapy is efficacious as part of the treatment regimen. Carboplatinum has a very limited role with significantly less efficacy when compared to cisplatinum based chemotherapy. The authors also found that patients with specific criteria, namely stage pT3 disease, lymph node positivity, and positive surgical margins (i.e. all portending high risk disease) may benefit from adjuvant chemotherapy. One basic question, based on our recent data defining relatively poor long term cancer-specific survival in those patients treated with high grade disease treated with nephroureterectomy, is whether a chemotherapeutic regimen including cisplatinum and gemcitabine should be employed neoadjuvantly. Similar to what is noted when employed prior to cystectomy, this pre-operative systemic treatment may improve pathologic staging and overall cancer-specific survival [35]. The increased risk of these systemic agents when renal function is compromised is commonly used as an argument against adjuvant therapy post nephrectomy. Employed on a neoadjuvant fashion, these agents have the added benefit of normal therapeutic dosing while the patient has maximal renal functional reserve [36].

In summary, ureteroscopic treatment of upper urinary tract urothelial tumors is efficacious in those patients presenting with low-grade disease, with similar cancer-specific and overall survival rates as compared to extirpative nephroureterectomy. Ureteroscopic intervention to mitigate severe symptoms in those patients with high-grade disease who are not candidates for nephroureterectomy also has merit, with the understanding that this is palliative, improving symptoms and lengthening survival, but not inhibiting progression in stage. Lastly, nephroureterectomy for high-grade disease has a relatively poor long-term cancer-specific survival as sole therapy. In those patients with high grade disease treated with nephroureterectomy there may be a role for either adjuvant or potentially neoadjuvant therapy to improve overall survival.

References

1. Huffman JL, Bagley DH, Lyon ES, et al. Endoscopic diagnosis and treatment of upper-tract urothelial tumors: a preliminary report. Cancer. 1985;55:1422–8.
2. Johnson GB, Portela D, Grasso M. Advanced ureteroscopy: wireless and sheathless. J Endourol. 2006;20(8):552–5.
3. Grasso M, Fraiman M, Levine M. Ureteropyeloscopic diagnosis and treatment of upper urinary tract urothelial malignancies. Urology. 1999;54(2):240–6.
4. Grasso M, Bagley DH. A 7.5/8.2 French actively deflectable, flexible ureteroscope: a new device for both diagnostic and therapeutic upper urinary tract endoscopy. Urology. 1994;43:435–41.
5. Johnson GB, Grasso M. Exaggerated primary endoscope deflection: initial clinical experience with prototypic flexible ureteroscopes: the first 115 procedures. BJU. 2003;93(1):109–14.
6. Bagley DH, Kulp DA, Bibbo M. Ureteroscopic biopsy optimized by cytopathologic techniques. J Urol. 1994;151:387A.
7. Abdel-Razzak OM, Ehya H, Cubler-Goodman A, Bagley DH. Ureteroscopic biopsy in the upper urinary tract. Urology. 1994;44:451–7.
8. Keeley FX, Kulp DA, Bibbo M, et al. Diagnostic accuracy of ureteroscopic biopsy in upper tract transitional cell carcinoma. J Urol. 1997;157:33–7.
9. Cutress ML, Stewart GD, Wells-Cole S, Phipps S, Thomas BG, Tolley DA. Long-term endoscopic management of upper tract urothelial carcinoma: 20-year single-centre experience. BJU Int. 2012;110(11):1608–17.
10. Daneshmand S, Quek ML, Huffman JL. Endoscopic management of upper urinary tract transitional cell carcinoma: long-term experience. Cancer. 2003;98:55–60.
11. Keeley Jr FX, Bibbo M, Bagley DH. Ureteroscopic treatment and surveillance of upper urinary tract transitional cell carcinoma. J Urol. 1997;157(5):1560–5.
12. Canfield SE, Dinney CP, Droller MJ. Surveillance and management of recurrence for upper tract transitional cell carcinoma. Urol Clin North Am. 2003;30(4):791–802.
13. Johnson G, Fraiman M, Grasso M. Broadening experience with the retrograde endoscopic management of upper urinary tract urothelial malignancies. BJU Int. 2005;95 Suppl 2:110–3.
14. Johnson GB, Grasso M. Ureteroscopic management of upper urinary tract transitional cell carcinoma. Curr Opin Urol. 2005;15(2):89–93.

15. Bagley DH, Grasso M. Ureteroscopic laser treatment of upper urinary tract neoplasms. World J Urol. 2010;28:143–9.

16. Schmeller NT, Hofstetter AG. Laser treatment of ureteral tumors. J Urol. 1989;141:840–3.

17. Floratos DL, de la Rosette JJ. Lasers in urology. BJU Int. 1999;84(2):204–11.

18. von Eschenbach A. Chapter 6: Superficial bladder cancer. In: Smith JA (editors) Lasers in urologic surgery. Yearbook Medical Publishing; 1989. The University of Michigan. p 57–66.

19. Ali Ansari M, Mohajerani E. Mechanisms of laser-tissue interaction: optical properties of tissue. J Lasers Med Sci. 2011;2(3):119–25.

20. Nargund VH, Tanabalan CK, Kabir MN. Management of non-muscle-invasive (superficial) bladder cancer. Semin Oncol. 2012;39(5):559–72.

21. Martinez-Pineiro JA, Garcia Matres MJ, Martinez-Pineiro L. Endourological treatment of upper tract urothelial carcinomas: analysis of a series of 59 tumors. J Urol. 1996;156(2 Pt 1):377–85.

22. Keeley Jr FX, Bagley DH. Adjuvant mitomycin C following endoscopic treatment of upper tract transitional cell carcinoma. J Urol. 1997;158(6):2074–7.

23. Aboumarzouk OM, Somani B, Ahmad S, Nabi G, Townell N, Kata SG. Mitomycin C instillation following ureterorenoscopic laser ablation of upper urinary tract carcinoma. Urol Ann. 2013;5(3):184–9.

24. Audenet F, Traxer O, Bensalah K, Rouprêt M. Upper urinary tract instillations in the treatment of urothelial carcinomas: a review of technical constraints and outcomes. World J Urol. 2013;31(1):45–52.

25. Cutress ML, Stewart GD, Zakikhani P, Phipps S, Thomas BG, Tolley DA. Ureteroscopic and percutaneous management of upper tract urothelial carcinoma (UTUC): systematic review. BJU Int. 2012;110(5):614–28.

26. Chew BH, Pautler SE, Denstedt JD. Percutaneous management of upper-tract transitional cell carcinoma. J Endourol. 2005;19(6):658–63.

27. Irwin BH, Berger AK, Brandina R, Stein R, Desai MM. Complex percutaneous resections for upper-tract urothelial carcinoma. J Endourol. 2010;24(3):367–70.

28. Rouprêt M, Traxer O, Tligui M, et al. Upper urinary tract transitional cell carcinoma: recurrence rate after percutaneous endoscopic resection. Eur Urol. 2007;51(3):709–14.

29. Grasso M, Fishman AI, Cohen J, Alexander B. Ureteroscopic and extirpative treatment of upper urinary tract urothelial carcinoma: a 15-year comprehensive review of 160 consecutive patients. BJU Int. 2012;110(11):1618–26.

30. van der Heijden AG, Witjes JA. Recurrence, progression, and follow-up in non–muscle-invasive bladder cancer. Eur Urol. 2009;8(Suppl):556–62.

31. Berger A, Haber GP, Kamoi K, et al. Laparoscopic radical nephroureterectomy for upper tract transitional cell carcinoma: oncological outcomes at 7 years. J Urol. 2008;180:849–54.

32. Elliott DS, Blute ML, Patterson DE, Bergstralh EJ, Segura JW. Long-term follow-up of endoscopically treated upper urinary tract transitional cell carcinoma. Urology. 1996;47(6):819–25.

33. Martínez-Piñeiro JA, García Matres MJ, Martínez-Piñeiro L. Endourological treatment of upper tract urothelial carcinomas: analysis of a series of 59 tumors. J Urol. 1996;156(2 Pt 1):377–85.

34. Leow JJ, Martin-Doyle W, Fay AP, Choueiri TK, Chang SL, Bellmunt J. A systematic review and meta-analysis of adjuvant and neoadjuvant chemotherapy for upper tract urothelial carcinoma. Eur Urol. 2014;66(3):529–41.

35. Grossman HB, Natale RB, Tangen CM, Speights VO, et al. Neoadjuvant chemotherapy plus cystectomy compared with cystectomy alone for locally advanced bladder cancer. N Engl J Med. 2003;349(9):859–66.

36. Porten S, Siefker-Radtke AO, Xiao L, et al. Neoadjuvant chemotherapy improves survival of patients with upper tract urothelial carcinoma. Cancer. 2014;120(12):1794–9.

Surgical Management of Upper Tract Urothelial Carcinoma– Open, Laparoscopic, and Robotic Approaches to Nephroureterectomy and Outcomes

5

Marc J. Mann, Costas D. Lallas, and Edouard J. Trabulsi

5.1 Introduction

It is estimated that upper tract urothelial carcinoma (UTUC) is a rare disease making up only 5–6 % of all urothelial malignancies, and occurs in only 1–4 people per 100,000 with a peak incidence in the 6th and 7th decades occurring in men more frequently than women [1]. Perhaps due to the rarity of incidence limiting research knowledge and the relatively aggressive nature at times of UTUC, surgical management of UTUC tends to be more aggressive than that of the lower tract. In order to adequately stage the disease, there is a heavy reliance on radiographic and visual imaging via ureteroscopy. The reason for this reliance on imaging and direct visualization is primarily due to the problem of obtaining tissue biopsies to accurately gauge depth of invasion. There are severe size limitations on the biopsy forceps, as it must fit through an ureteroscope. As a result reliance has been on grading of the cellular atypia rather than the clinical T stage of the disease. Indeed, studies have shown direct correlation with tumor grade and degree of invasion on final pathologic analysis although under-grading occurs up to 25 % of the time [2]. Anatomically, there are relatively thinner layers of tissue between the surface of then urothelium to the surrounding adventitia for the development of locally advanced disease in the kidney and ureter, as compared to the urothelium in the bladder. This causes a higher risk of each lesion to progress. Furthermore, as opposed to cases of bladder cancer with superficial high-grade disease, where one has the options to treat with intravesical washings of chemotherapies and immunotherapies via a catheter, in UTUC it is necessary to use sedation or anesthesia to cystoscopically place a ureteral catheter or to percutaneously place a nephrostomy tube. Despite the invasive nature of applying the treatment, and limitations due to natural peristalsis, utilization of various methods of renal pelvic and ureteral irrigation with BCG is an option for select patients with CIS of the upper tracts [3, 4]. As organ-sparing options with intraluminal chemotherapies are limited, and the relatively thinner barriers for tumor progression compared to lower tract urothelial carcinoma (LTUC); the gold standard for treatment of UTUC continues to be radical nephroureterectomy (RNU). In this chapter

M.J. Mann, MD • C.D. Lallas, MD
Department of Urology,
Thomas Jefferson University, 1025 Walnut Street,
Philadelphia, PA 19107, USA

E.J. Trabulsi, MD, FACS (✉)
Department of Urology,
Kimmel Cancer Center, Sidney Kimmel Medical
College, Thomas Jefferson University,
1025 Walnut Street, Philadelphia, PA 19107, USA
e-mail: Edouard.Trabulsi@jefferson.edu

© Springer International Publishing Switzerland 2015
M. Grasso III, D.H. Bagley (eds.), *Upper Urinary Tract Urothelial Carcinoma*,
DOI 10.1007/978-3-319-13869-5_5

we will discuss the surgical management of UTUC as well as innovations in the surgical approach and current controversies.

5.2 Indications for RNU or Partial Ureterectomy

Conservative management of UTUC via endoscopic laser ablation, or intraluminal chemotherapy, is indicated in cases of low-grade/low-volume tumor burden disease. However, in many cases, even when the tumor is low-grade, the volume or bulk of disease can overwhelm the ability to of intraluminal chemotherapy or laser ablation to manage, surgical management is indicated. Furthermore, if the tumor is high-grade surgical management is indicated [5]. This is true even if there are suspicious lymph nodes on imaging as well [6]. There is little evidence to support performing a RNU in the presence of proven metastatic lymph nodes, as survival is poor, however, after treatment response with neoadjuvant chemotherapy, it can be considered [6]. In instances of proven or metastatic disease chemotherapy and radiation should be encouraged. However, in clinically localized disease, the gold standard of surgical management consists of removal of the affected kidney and ureter en bloc with a bladder cuff around the ipsilateral ureteral orifice.

It is important to be cognizant that as a result of the loss of 50 % of a patient's nephrons from the RNU, the choice of chemotherapeutics and need for substitution of treatments can decrease survival and limit the efficacy of chemotherapies. Radical removal of nephrons via nephrectomy has been proven to decrease overall survival in renal cell carcinoma [7]. In addition, renal failure as a result of renal surgery or otherwise, is associated with accelerated atherosclerosis and concomitant increase in cardiovascular morbidity [8, 9]. As a result, there is renewed interest in nephron-sparing surgical treatments for UTUC such as partial ureterectomy [10]. In addition, the development of minimally invasive surgical techniques of laparoscopy and robotic-

assisted laparoscopic surgery have both made significant inroads in the treatment algorithm for UTUC and will be discussed as well in this chapter.

5.3 Open Radical Nephroureterectomy and Treatment of the Bladder Cuff

Open RNU is the radical removal of the kidney, ureter, and bladder cuff and is the gold standard for treatment for clinically localized high grade UTUC [11]. The decision tree of the type of procedure begins with approach of open, laparoscopic or robotic-assisted laparoscopic. In this segment, we will describe the outcomes and considerations of the open approach. The next decision point is the application of a lymphadenectomy and/or extent of it. The application and utility of lymphadenectomy will be described in a separate section below. Finally, we will discuss here the various approaches to the removal of the bladder cuff around the insertion of the ureter into the bladder urothelium.

There are a number of incisions that can be made for a RNU can. One can perform a two-incision technique, whereupon the kidney is dissected free from the vascular hilum and the upper ureter via a flank incision and a subsequent Gibson incision for freeing the rest of the ureter up to the bladder enabling the completion of the entire procedure in an extraperitoneal fashion. Alternatively, one can perform the same procedure completely from a pubic to sternum midline incision violating the peritoneum, but allowing for fantastic exposure and access to all major vessels after incising along the white line of Toldt and reflecting the colon (and duodenum if on the right side). Choice of incision tends to be surgeon preference and comfort with considerations for the particular surgical history and tumor anatomy of the individual patient.

Conversely, the decision of the approach to the bladder cuff does have significant oncological implications. In a retrospective Canadian study pooling results from 10 institutions, 5-year survival for RNU has been shown to be 46–30 % varying primarily with the approach to the bladder cuff removed with the specimen [12]. There are three approaches that can be taken to the distal ureter. It can be removed intravesically whereupon an extraperitoneal open incision is made in the anterior bladder after the kidney and ureter have been dissected free and the ureteral orifice (UO) is incised from inside the bladder until free altogether. The intravesical resection of the bladder cuff was associated with the best disease-free survival of 46.3 % at 5 years. There is also the extravesical approach whereupon the ureter is dissected free through the detrusor until completely free, this approach was found to have a disease-free survival (DFS) of 38.5 % at 5 years. Finally, there is the endoscopic approach, whereupon after freeing the kidney and ureter up to the detrusor the ureteral orifice is then incised with a Collins knife or an electrocautery knife or resected with a loop and then closed from within the peritoneal cavity. The distal ureter has been described as closed using an endoloop to prevent tumor seeding. This approach was found to have an 11.9 % disease-free survival at 5 years. This data is consistent with older literature using the SEER database and other retrospective reviews, as there have been no randomized studies performed to date. The evidence seems to support intravesical or extravesical approaches to the bladder cuff in open RNU [13–16].

Since up to 34 % of patients can recur after RNU with tumors in the bladder, studies have analyzed perioperative treatment of the bladder with chemotherapeutic washing at time of RNU [17]. The OMDIT-C British trial published in 2011 of patients with UTUC randomized to instillation of one dose of Mitomycin C for prevention of bladder tumor recurrence after RNU, found a decreased incidence of bladder recurrence in analysis by treatment of 16 % (compared to 27 %) at 1 year follow up [18]. While it is not by any means standard of care, it is an option to strongly consider for tumor recurrences in the bladder after RNU.

5.4 Laparoscopic Nephroureterectomy

The indications for performance of a laparoscopic RNU (LRNU) are the same as that for open RNU, however, the patient must be able to tolerate 15 mmHg pneumoperitoneum from a cardiopulmonary anesthesia stand-point. The benefits of minimally invasive surgery are much the same here in terms of decreased blood loss, cosmesis of smaller incisions and quicker convalescence, much as they are in comparison of open and laparoscopic radical nephrectomy. The positioning and port placement for LRNU can be the same as that for a laparoscopic radical nephrectomy with or without a hand-port or an additional 12-mm port in either the right or left lower quadrant to assist in the dissection of the distal ureter. There are various iterations of positioning and port placement for laparoscopic radical nephrectomy. We place the patient in a modified flank position with a 10-pound sand bag underneath the ipsilateral flank and the patient secured to the bed with straps loosely over the legs (which are elevated on pillows) and tightly across the hips and chest. For trocar placement, we prefer the use of a medial 12 mm camera port placement approximately 2 cm superior to the umbilicus and 2 cm lateral to midline or just lateral to rectus abdominus with two working ports in the mid clavicular line approximately 12 cm apart centered on the camera port with the superior port being a 5 mm and the inferior port being a 12 mm. An additional 5 mm port may be placed for liver retraction as well. A hand port can either be placed in the midline infra-umbilically or via an ipsilateral Gibson incision. If intention is for a purely laparoscopic approach, after the kidney and the ureter is dissected down past the superior vesicle artery, the bladder can then be opened at the dome and the ureteral orifice is ligated and then dissected free with a bladder cuff intravesically (or extravesically) until completely freed. The specimen is always removed in a bag to prevent tumor seeding [19]. Alternatively, some may prefer to combine laparoscopic dissection of the kidney and bladder with an extraperitoneal/intravesical bladder cuff to reduce the theoretically risk of peritoneal tumor seeding.

Outcomes from LRNU with and without hand-assistance have been well documented. Berger published in 2008 outcomes for LRNU including up to 7 years of median follow up with 50 % overall survival (OAS) 72 % cancer-specific survival (CSS) and 36 % recurrence-free survival (RFS) [20]. This data is consistent with other long-term data published previously in open and laparoscopic surgeries [21, 22]. However, in regards to higher stage disease, outcomes data comparing open to laparoscopic procedures remain conflicting [14, 15, 23–25]. At this point in time it is safe to declare that LRNU has similar outcomes to the open approach in lower stage disease, and this may be true for locally advanced as well, however, further study is necessary to elucidate that point.

5.5 Robotic Nephroureterectomy

Indications for robotic-assisted laparoscopic RNU (RALNU) are the same as for LRNU. The trifecta combination of limited work-hours on residents and the time intensity of laparoscopic training with increased mobility of the DaVinci Xi Robotic surgical platform has led to our expectation that the application of robotic technology to nephroureterectomy will increase in popularity. We expect this confluence of factors to cause a relative increase in the numbers of procedures performed due to both surgeon skill set as well as by patient demand in the near future. In fact, even prior to the development of the DaVinci Xi platform, using the older DaVinci systems, RALNU had already been described first by Nanigian and then altered by Park to alleviate the need for repositioning for the bladder cuff [26]. The benefits of robotic surgery over laparoscopic surgery for UTUC remain primarily in the 7° of freedom, 90° of articulation with motion scaling and tremor reduction that the robotic system offers and relatively lower threshold of training for surgeons to obtain for competency. Port placement has yet to be standardized, and is likely to change as the DaVinci Xi system becomes more popular as the camera and arms can be interchangeably placed through ports, but for the Si and earlier models, the ports are arranged the same as for a Nephrectomy with an extra infraumbilical midline 12 mm port for the 8 mm robotic arm trocar to get placed into for the bladder cuff.

Outcomes data is still young for outcomes of RALNU, however, perioperative outcomes appear to be on par with outcomes of LRNU [27, 28]. A retrospective review of 11 patients underwent RALNU and after a mean follow-up of 30 months, only 1 patient had a recurrence for a RFS of 91 % at 2.5 years [29]. While the very limited available evidence is encouraging, studies with significantly greater numbers and longer follow up must be performed before any conclusions can be made about this very exciting area of innovation.

5.6 Partial Ureterectomy

As a result of the earlier mentioned concern about loss of nephrons leading to a higher risk of mortality from cardiovascular complications, there has been increased pressure to apply more renal-preserving treatment approaches with increased volumes of lower-grade disease treated with intraluminal therapies as well as endoscopic laser ablations. In addition, more interest in distal or partial ureterectomy has occurred. Indications for partial or distal ureterectomy include functionally solitary or solitary kidney, and bilateral disease. In cases where the tumor is localized to a single segment, especially the distal segment. Segmental ureterectomy can also be considered when there is a significant likelihood of higher T-stage disease and adjuvant or salvage chemotherapy is likely to require nephron-sparing treatment. The procedure can be performed open, laparoscopic or robotically [30, 31]. Depending on the area excised, the drainage can be reconstructed with a Boari Flap and or a Psoas hitch, an end to end spatulated ureteroureterostomy, a ureteroneocystostomy, appendiceal substitution, autotransplantation as well as others [32–34].

Outcomes of a study reviewing SEER data of 569 patients who underwent partial ureterectomy compared to 1,222 patients who underwent RNU with a bladder cuff showed no significant differences in the 77.6 % 5-year CSS in multivariate analysis by surgical modality [35]. These results are consistent when compared to multinstitutional data on RNU, as well as in more recent comparisons of partial ureterectomy [36–38]. The current available literature all consists of retrospective reviews again likely including a patient selection bias, indicating that in select cases this can be an excellent treatment option.

5.7 Lymphadenectomy During RNU

The evaluation of regional and distant lymph nodes (LNs) is imperative in the staging of cancers. This is often performed clinically preoperatively with radiographic imaging. However, when performing a RNU or segmental ureterectomy for UTUC, the evaluation of the evaluation of the LNs is critical as it is estimated that 20–40 % will develop LN involvement due to the relatively thin walls and variable copious lymphatic drainage [37, 39–42]. It has been well documented that in patients with muscle invasive urothelial cell carcinoma of the bladder performance of a lympadenectomy (LAD) leads to identification of more positive nodes in patients with positive nodes. While it is unclear if there is any survival benefit, but rather just a "Roy Rogers Phenomenon," where the high risk patients do worse as their positive LNs are identified and up-staged, and the LN negative patients are down-staged. This question is currently being answered by a Phase III randomized clinical trial for bladder cancer [43].

Regarding UTUC, the question of whether the benefit of the performance of a lymphadenectomy (LAD) is prognostic or therapeutic remains somewhat controversial. There are several issues with determining the answer to this question. Performance of an LAD along with the RNU for UTUC is widely variable making consist operative data sets difficult to find and interpret. There is also a variable lymphatic drainage based on the location of the tumor in the upper tract, and there are no clearly defined borders or templates regarding the correct LNs that require excision [41, 42]. There is no well-defined number of lymph nodes that are required to be removed. It is well documented that pathologic node-status strongly predicts outcomes with node-negative disease 2–3 times worse [44, 45]. As a result of the benefit achieved by node-negative disease on pathology, some urge performance of LAD in order to remove any microscopic metastatic disease that may be in those nodes that may offer this survival benefit.

However, what is an adequate LAD? Based on studies on of the relationship between area of tumor and area of positive lymph nodes, Kondo et al. suggested that area which an LAD should be done should be based on level of tumor location. For UTUC of the renal pelvis and kidney LAD should be performed on the ipsilateral perihilar and for tumors on the right, paracaval, retrocaval and inter-aortocaval, and on the left para-aortic from the level of the hilum to the level of the inferior mesenteric artery. For UTUC of the upper 2/3 of the ureter, the borders of the LAD are the same except it is progressed from the level of the hilum down to the aortic bifurcation. Finally, for UTUC in the lower 1/3 of the ureter, one should perform an LAD of the ipsilateral common iliac artery and vein with the ureter as the medial border and the side wall as the lateral border to the node of cloquet as well as down into the obturator fossa and internal iliac vessels. Kondo based this template upon where at least 10 % of the metastatic lymph nodes were found for each level with UTUC [46, 47]. This template would offer very high yield results, although it has yet to be validated from larger and multi-institutional studies and in addition, missing 10 % of metastatic disease results in those patients being under-staged.

At this point in time, this anatomical dissection template is not universally accepted. Some studies have suggested that eight is the optimal number of LNs removed in order to detect the presence or absence of metastatic disease [5]. Others argue that what is necessary for ideal outcome, there must be a LN density (percent of tumor-bearing LNs of all LNs excised) of 20 % or more to show poorer survival [48]. Although, some authors argue that these results are really predicated on the pT stage of the disease with only stage pT2+ actually receive a benefit form performance of an LAD [49].

The likelihood of there being a benefit from removal of potentially microscopically metastatic (negative on pathological examination) lymph nodes is augmented by a number of studies comparing the results from retrospective reviews of patients who had a lymph node dissection and were pN0 (LAD performed and all nodes negative) to those who were pNx (LAD not performed) to those who were pN+(LAD performed and LN found to be positive). Studies all support that both pNx and PN0 are superior to pN+, however, results conflict, if pNo is superior to pNx. The most recently published study by Ouzzane et al. on 714 patients from 1995 to 2010 who underwent RNU for UTUC, found no significant benefit to performance of a LAD in LN negative patients. However, this result from Ouzzane conflicts with prior studies performed by Roscigno which found a step-wise improvement in survival based on the stratification of LN status from pN0 to pNx to pN+ (71 % to 69 % to 35 % p=0.032) [5, 50]. The loss of significance in LN status between these studies is very possibly the results of progressively improved imaging better able to identify suspicious LNs, which may lead surgeons to decide whether it is necessary to perform an LAD or not. Thus, the theoretical survival benefit in RNU of performing a LAD may in fact, be the result of poor selection bias that has improved with enhanced imaging techniques and interpretations. As time passes neo-adjuvant and adjuvant chemotherapy are likely to be used more efficaciously and imaging quality continues to improve, we may find that the micro-metastases that were supposedly treated by the LAD therapeutically become treated by the chemotherapy.

At this point in time, the National Cancer Institute holds the position that performance of a LAD may offer prognostic information and minimal if any therapeutic information. The National Cancer Center Network states a LAD should be performed for high-grade or high-volume or invasive tumors. The European Urological Association's guidelines from 2013 gives a grade C to the evidence, but supports performance of a LAD for invasive tumors.

Conclusions

RNU remains the gold standard treatment for high-grade or high-volume UTUC unable to be managed endoscopically. LRNU appears to have almost equivalent outcomes as open RNU however as fewer work hours limit the amount of time residents may spend training their laparoscopic skills and due to the ease of the robotic platform, it may be that we may find this level of skill erodes with time. Furthermore, as robotic surgical experience grows for RNU and the Xi DaVinci platform disseminates, we hypothesize that RALNU will become more popular and that studies will likely show equivalence to open after experiences with it matures. With the ever-greater push to spare more nephrons, in select cases performance of a segmental ureterectomy is a viable option. Finally, performance of an LAD is encouraged in cases of invasive tumors, especially when imaging identifies suspicious LNs, however, it is unclear if the number of LNs, or LN density or LN template is the best way to approach it.

References

1. Roupret M, et al. European guidelines for the diagnosis and management of upper urinary tract urothelial cell carcinomas: 2011 update. Eur Urol. 2011;59(4):584–94.
2. Yamany T, et al. Ureterorenoscopy for upper tract urothelial carcinoma: how often are we missing lesions? Urology. 2015;85(2):311–5.
3. Maurice MJ, et al. Retrograde chemoinfusion of the upper tract: standardizing the delivery of topical adjuvant therapy. J Endourol. 2013;27(5):540–4.
4. Pollard ME, et al. Comparison of 3 upper tract anti-carcinogenic agent delivery techniques in an ex vivo porcine model. Urology 2013;82(6):1451.e1–6.
5. Roscigno M, et al. Assessment of the minimum number of lymph nodes needed to detect lymph node invasion at radical nephroureterectomy in patients with upper tract urothelial cancer. Urology. 2009;74(5):1070–4.
6. Yang D, et al. Effect of lymph node dissection on the outcomes of upper tract urothelial carcinomas: a meta-analysis. Expert Rev Anticancer Ther. 2014;14(6):667–75.
7. Badalato GM, et al. Survival after partial and radical nephrectomy for the treatment of stage T1bN0M0 renal cell carcinoma (RCC) in the USA: a propensity scoring approach. BJU Int. 2012;109(10):1457–62.
8. Go AS, et al. Chronic kidney disease and the risks of death, cardiovascular events, and hospitalization. N Engl J Med. 2004;351(13):1296–305.
9. Weight CJ, et al. Nephrectomy induced chronic renal insufficiency is associated with increased risk

of cardiovascular death and death from any cause in patients with localized cT1b renal masses. J Urol. 2010;183(4):1317–23.

10. Smith P, Mandel J, Raman JD. Conservative nephron-sparing treatment of upper-tract tumors. Curr Urol Rep. 2013;14(2):102–8.

11. Roupret M, et al. European guidelines on upper tract urothelial carcinomas: 2013 update. Eur Urol. 2013;63(6):1059–71.

12. Kapoor A, et al. The impact of method of distal ureter management during radical nephroureterectomy on tumour recurrence. Can Urol Assoc J. 2014;8(11–12):E845–52.

13. Xylinas E, et al. Impact of distal ureter management on oncologic outcomes following radical nephroureterectomy for upper tract urothelial carcinoma. Eur Urol. 2014;65(1):210–7.

14. Seisen T, et al. A systematic review and meta-analysis of clinicopathologic factors linked to intravesical recurrence after radical nephroureterectomy to treat upper tract urothelial carcinoma. Eur Urol. 2015;67:1122–33.

15. Fairey AS, et al. Comparison of oncological outcomes for open and laparoscopic radical nephroureterectomy: results from the Canadian Upper Tract Collaboration. BJU Int. 2013;112(6):791–7.

16. Matin SF, Gill IS. Recurrence and survival following laparoscopic radical nephroureterectomy with various forms of bladder cuff control. J Urol. 2005;173(2):395–400.

17. Hirano D, et al. Intravesical recurrence after surgical management of urothelial carcinoma of the upper urinary tract. Urol Int. 2012;89(1):71–7.

18. O'Brien T, et al. Prevention of bladder tumours after nephroureterectomy for primary upper urinary tract urothelial carcinoma: a prospective, multicentre, randomised clinical trial of a single postoperative intravesical dose of mitomycin C (the ODMIT-C Trial). Eur Urol. 2011;60(4):703–10.

19. Naderi N, et al. Port site metastasis after laparoscopic nephro-ureterectomy for transitional cell carcinoma. Eur Urol. 2004;46(4):440–1.

20. Berger A, et al. Laparoscopic radical nephroureterectomy for upper tract transitional cell carcinoma: oncological outcomes at 7 years. J Urol. 2008;180(3):849–54; discussion 854.

21. Muntener M, et al. Long-term oncologic outcome after laparoscopic radical nephroureterectomy for upper tract transitional cell carcinoma. Eur Urol. 2007;51(6):1639–44.

22. Brown JA, et al. Hand-assisted laparoscopic nephroureterectomy: analysis of distal ureterectomy technique, margin status, and surgical outcomes. Urology. 2005;66(6):1192–6.

23. Simone G, et al. Laparoscopic versus open nephroureterectomy: perioperative and oncologic outcomes from a randomised prospective study. Eur Urol. 2009;56(3):520–6.

24. Walton TJ, et al. Oncological outcomes after laparoscopic and open radical nephroureterectomy: results from an international cohort. BJU Int. 2011;108(3):406–12.

25. Ariane MM, et al. Assessment of oncologic control obtained after open versus laparoscopic nephroureterectomy for upper urinary tract urothelial carcinomas (UUT-UCs): results from a large French multicenter collaborative study. Ann Surg Oncol. 2012;19(1):301–8.

26. Nanigian DK, Smith W, Ellison LM. Robot-assisted laparoscopic nephroureterectomy. J Endourol. 2006;20(7):463–5; discussion 465–6.

27. Marshall S, Stifelman M. Robot-assisted surgery for the treatment of upper urinary tract urothelial carcinoma. Urol Clin North Am. 2014;41(4):521–37.

28. Pugh J, et al. Perioperative outcomes of robot-assisted nephroureterectomy for upper urinary tract urothelial carcinoma: a multi-institutional series. BJU Int. 2013;112(4):E295–300.

29. Eandi JA, et al. Oncologic outcomes for complete robot-assisted laparoscopic management of upper-tract transitional cell carcinoma. J Endourol. 2010;24(6):969–75.

30. Stravodimos KG, et al. Distal ureterectomy techniques in laparoscopic and robot-assisted nephroureterectomy: Updated review. Urol Ann. 2015;7(1):8–16.

31. Uberoi J, et al. Robot-assisted laparoscopic distal ureterectomy and ureteral reimplantation with psoas hitch. J Endourol. 2007;21(4):368–73; discussion 372–3.

32. Lieber MM, Lupu AN. High grade invasive ureteral transitional cell carcinoma with a congenital solitary kidney: long-term survival after ureterectomy and radiation therapy. J Urol. 1978;120(3):368–9.

33. Ashley MS, Daneshmand S. Re: Appendiceal substitution following right proximal ureter injury. Int Braz J Urol. 2009;35(1):90–1.

34. Pettersson S, et al. Treatment of urothelial tumors of the upper urinary tract by nephroureterectomy, renal autotransplantation, and pyelocystostomy. Cancer. 1984;54(3):379–86.

35. Lughezzani G, et al. Nephroureterectomy and segmental ureterectomy in the treatment of invasive upper tract urothelial carcinoma: a population-based study of 2299 patients. Eur J Cancer. 2009;45(18):3291–7.

36. Colin P, et al. Comparison of oncological outcomes after segmental ureterectomy or radical nephroureterectomy in urothelial carcinomas of the upper urinary tract: results from a large French multicentre study. BJU Int. 2012;110(8):1134–41.

37. Margulis V, et al. Outcomes of radical nephroureterectomy: a series from the Upper Tract Urothelial Carcinoma Collaboration. Cancer. 2009;115(6):1224–33.

38. Simhan J, et al. Nephron-sparing management vs radical nephroureterectomy for low- or moderate-grade, low-stage upper tract urothelial carcinoma. BJU Int. 2014;114(2):216–20.

39. Batata MA, et al. Primary carcinoma of the ureter: a prognostic study. Cancer. 1975;35(6):1626–32.

40. Whitlock GF, Mc DJ, Cook EN. Primary carcinoma of the ureter: a pathologic and prognostic study. J Urol. 1955;73(2):245–53.

41. Kondo T, et al. Primary site and incidence of lymph node metastases in urothelial carcinoma of upper urinary tract. Urology. 2007;69(2):265–9.

42. Secin FP, et al. Evaluation of regional lymph node dissection in patients with upper urinary tract urothelial cancer. Int J Urol. 2007;14(1):26–32.

43. Gakis G, et al. ICUD-EAU International Consultation on Bladder Cancer 2012: radical cystectomy and bladder preservation for muscle-invasive urothelial carcinoma of the bladder. Eur Urol. 2013;63(1):45–57.

44. Cha EK, et al. Predicting clinical outcomes after radical nephroureterectomy for upper tract urothelial carcinoma. Eur Urol. 2012;61(4):818–25.

45. Favaretto RL, et al. The effect of tumor location on prognosis in patients treated with radical nephroureterectomy at Memorial Sloan-Kettering Cancer Center. Eur Urol. 2010;58(4):574–80.

46. Kondo T, Tanabe K. Role of lymphadenectomy in the management of urothelial carcinoma of the bladder and the upper urinary tract. Int J Urol. 2012;19(8):710–21.

47. Abe T, et al. Outcome of regional lymphadenectomy in accordance with primary tumor location on laparoscopic nephroureterectomy for urothelial carcinoma of the upper urinary tract: a prospective study. J Endourol. 2015;29:304–9.

48. Mason RJ, et al. The contemporary role of lymph node dissection during nephroureterectomy in the management of upper urinary tract urothelial carcinoma: the Canadian experience. Urology. 2012;79(4):840–5.

49. Burger M, et al. No overt influence of lymphadenectomy on cancer-specific survival in organ-confined versus locally advanced upper urinary tract urothelial carcinoma undergoing radical nephroureterectomy: a retrospective international, multi-institutional study. World J Urol. 2011;29(4):465–72.

50. Ouzzane A, et al. The impact of lymph node status and features on oncological outcomes in urothelial carcinoma of the upper urinary tract (UTUC) treated by nephroureterectomy. World J Urol. 2013;31(1):189–97.

Surveillance After Treatment for Upper Tract Transitional Cell Carcinoma

6

Michael J. Conlin and Brian D. Duty

6.1 Introduction

Urothelial tumors involving the upper urinary tract are uncommon, accounting for approximately 5 % of all renal tumors and 5 % of transitional cell carcinomas [12]. Over the past two decades the incidence of renal pelvic tumors has been relatively stable but there has been a marginal increase in ureteral cancers [19].

Review of the National Cancer Database between 1993 and 2005 revealed a stage migration with a greater proportion of individuals being diagnosed with non-muscle invasive disease [6]. Despite this, disease specific survival has not changed significantly over the past 20 years, which may be accounted for by the increased incidence of high-grade tumors [19].

Age at diagnosis has increased over time with a peak incidence now occurring between ages 75 and 79 [24]. As a result, more patients undergoing nephroureterectomy will likely develop chronic renal insufficiency, placing them at increased risk of all-cause mortality and cardiovascular events [8]. Additionally, the 5-year life expectancy of a septuagenarian on hemodialysis is only 10 % [18].

M.J. Conlin, MD, MCR, FACS (✉) • B.D. Duty, MD
Department of Urology, Oregon Health & Science University, OHSU Center for Health and Healing, Oregon Health and Science University,
3303 SW Bond Ave., 10th floor CH10u,
Portland, OR 97239, USA
e-mail: conlinm@ohsu.edu

Once reserved for strictly imperative indications (e.g., solitary kidney, bilateral tumors, prohibitive comorbidities), endoscopic treatment of upper tract tumors has increased due to refinements in equipment, technique and the improved understanding of the deleterious impact of chronic renal insufficiency. Patients treated endoscopically are at high risk for recurrence (23–60 %) with large, multifocal and high-grade lesions being more likely to recur [5]. Fortunately successful detection and treatment of recurrences is possible with diligent surveillance. Chen and Bagley reported their experience with ureteroscopic treatment of low-grade upper tract transitional cell carcinoma in 23 patients with normal contralateral kidneys. Sixty-five percent of these patients had multiple recurrences which were all successfully treated ureteroscopically. At the time of their last follow-up, 65 % were free of ipsilateral disease, and none of the patients had experienced disease progression [4].

Because upper tract tumors have such a high recurrence rate surveillance is an absolutely critical, but challenging, component of any endoscopic treatment strategy. More than merely identifying recurrent disease, surveillance guides treatment decisions. Further management is governed by the size, location, multiplicity, grade and stage of recurrent lesions.

In contrast to bladder cancer, surveillance of the upper tracts is not amenable to a quick office-based procedure. This is particularly true for

M. Grasso III, D.H. Bagley (eds.), *Upper Urinary Tract Urothelial Carcinoma*,
DOI 10.1007/978-3-319-13869-5_6

individuals with urinary diversions who develop an upper tract recurrence following radical cystectomy. This chapter will review surveillance techniques and provide recommendations based upon the limited published studies/guidelines.

6.2 Tools for Upper Tract Surveillance

A number of tools are available to detect and stage tumor recurrences. These factors include cytology, retrograde ureteropyelography, computed tomography (CT) ureteropyelography, and direct ureteroscopic inspection.

New bladder tumors can develop in up to 35 % of patients with upper tract transitional cell carcinoma regardless of how they are treated [3, 4, 7, 9, 10, 15, 16, 17, 25, 26]. Therefore, cystoscopy must be included in any upper tract surveillance regimen. During cystoscopy, retrograde ureteropyelograms can be performed to evaluate the upper tract. Retrograde ureteropyelography has a number of advantages. It can be performed without anesthesia either in clinic or during an ambulatory surgical procedure. Additionally, it allows for upper tract screening in patients who cannot receive intravenous contrast, such as patients with renal insufficiency.

Whether retrograde ureteropyelography alone is sufficient as an upper tract screening tool (with regard to cancer-specific and overall survival) is a matter of debate. However, it has been shown that ureteroscopy is more sensitive than retrograde ureteropyelography in detecting recurrent small upper tract tumors [15, 26]. Level four data does support that cytology and pyelography alone are insufficient surveillance modalities. A study of 88 surveillance ureteroscopies performed on 23 patients who had undergone endoscopic management of low-grade upper tract urothelial tumors found that bladder cytology and retrograde pyelography had a sensitivity of only 50 % and 72 %, respectively [4]. The sensitivity of ureteroscopic biopsy was 93 %. A limitation of this study was the absence of patients with high-grade lesions. However,

barring imperative indications, most patients with high-grade tumors are best managed with extirpative therapy.

In the past, radiologic studies (CT, excretory urography, retrograde studies) were relied upon to evaluate the upper urinary tracts in patients with urothelial tumors. Improvements in ureteroscopic instrumentation and technique have greatly enhanced the safety and efficacy of diagnostic ureteroscopy. Upper urinary tract filling defects seen on excretory or retrograde urography can often be fully evaluated with direct ureteroscopic visual inspection [2]. Ureteroscopic appearance of upper tract urothelial carcinoma is similar to the familiar cystoscopic appearance of bladder-based urothelial carcinoma. Low-grade urothelial tumors have a typical papillary appearance (Fig. 6.1). Higher grade tumors can be more sessile and at times necrotic appearing. Although upper urinary tract transitional cell carcinoma can often be identified by direct ureteroscopic inspection, this should not be the sole basis of diagnosis. When evaluating any soft-tissue lesion concerning for urothelial cancer, the diagnosis should be based on visual appearance, cytologic evaluation, and biopsy [15].

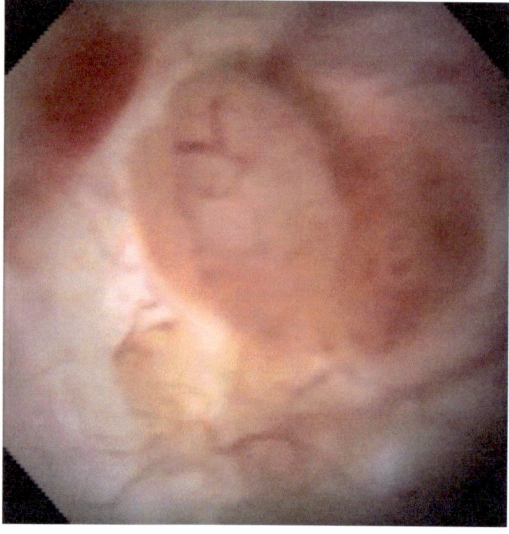

Fig. 6.1 Typical ureteroscopic appearance of a small papillary low grade tumor in the renal pelvis

Accurate staging of upper urinary tract transitional cell carcinoma is challenging. CT evaluation alone has been shown inadequate for accurate staging, and the underlying ureteral musculature can seldom be safely sampled ureteroscopically. Fortunately, stage and grade correlate closely, allowing grade to help guide treatment options [15]. While cytology is specific, it is less sensitive because most low-grade lesions will be missed. Higher grade transitional cell carcinoma lesions are more likely to provide positive cytologic findings as the tumor cells have lost their cell-cell adhesion capabilities and demonstrate more easily identifiable morphologic changes. Direct ureteroscopic biopsy is highly sensitive but less specific. Thus, cytology and biopsy are complementary tools in diagnosing and grading these tumors.

Minimizing ureteral trauma during ureteroscopy is important to maintain excellent visibility, diminish trauma related erroneous lesions, and to decrease the risk of tumor seeding during ureteroscopy. Ureteroscope outer diameter has decreased over time, which has improved our ability to insert the ureteroscope without prior ureteral dilation [11]. This is critical because prestenting or ureteral dilation at the time of surgery creates iatrogenic trauma that can be difficult to distinguish from recurrent disease, particularly carcinoma in situ. As the invasiveness of ureteroscopy decreases, there will be fewer reasons to rely on radiologic studies when one can safely inspect and sample the urothelium of the upper urinary tract.

Patients with significant comorbidities make ureteroscopic inspection a higher risk endeavor. For these patients, retrograde ureteropyelography alone may be a reasonable alternative. In these patients, ureteroscopy can be reserved for further investigation of significant filling defects. There are no data showing improved survival with one screening method over another. Although it is known that small tumors will be missed with retrograde ureteropyelograms alone, it is not unclear if delaying treatment of these small recurrences until they are large enough to be detected on retrograde ureteropyelography will result in any additional harm to the patient. Nevertheless, direct ureteroscopic inspection is favored over retrograde pyelography and voided cytology in patients without prohibitive comorbidities.

6.3 Surveillance Protocols

As detailed, multiple surveillance options exist following endoscopic treatment of upper tract tumors. Bagley and colleagues sent a survey to members of the Society of Urologic Oncology, Endourological Society, and American Urological Association regarding treatment and surveillance strategies for upper tract tumors [21]. Seventy percent of respondents performed surveillance ureteroscopy. The remainder used excretory urography or retrograde pyelography without upper tract endoscopy. Time to initial surveillance ureteroscopy was split evenly between 3- and 6-months. None of the responders relied entirely on urinary markers.

At present there are no detailed, evidence-based guidelines on the ideal surveillance protocol, which is highlighted by the wide variety of practice patterns. One of the most detailed surveillance protocols has been outlined by the Jefferson University group [21]. Their institutional protocol consists of cystoscopy, retrograde pyelography and ureteroscopy every 3 months until the patient is disease free. Office cystoscopy is then performed at 3, 9, 15, and 21 months. Ureteroscopy in the operating room is performed at the 6, 12, 18 and 24 month mark. After the first 2 years, cystoscopy is performed every 6 months and ureteroscopy annually.

The American Urological Association has not released any guidelines pertaining to the management of upper tract urothelial tumors. The National Comprehensive Cancer Network (NCCN) Bladder Cancer Guidelines do provide specific management recommendations for upper tract tumors but their surveillance recommendations are limited (NCCN guidelines). The guidelines recommend follow-up ureteroscopy and upper tract imaging (intravenous pyelography, retrograde pyelogram, CT or magnetic resonance urography) at 3–12 month intervals. Decreased surveillance frequency over time for patients without evidence of recurrence is not addressed.

The European Association of Urology has published guidelines on urothelial tumors of the upper tract [23]. Following endoscopic treatment, the Guidelines recommend performing urinary cytology and CT urography at 3 and 6 months then annually for at least 5 years. Cystoscopy, ureteroscopy and in situ cytology is also performed at the 3 and 6 month mark, then every 6 months for 2 years, then yearly.

A summary of the two available sets of recommendations for surveillance of patients following treatment of upper tract urothelial carcinoma is presented in Table 6.1.

Our recommended surveillance protocol algorithm for these patients is presented in Fig. 6.2. In our protocol, the frequency of cystoscopy and upper tract imaging is based on the treatment of patients with low grade urothelial carcinoma, as this will make up the majority of patients treated endoscopically. There are very few recommendations in the NCCN and EAU guidelines regarding surveillance following nephroureterectomy. In the absence of any specific guidance, we recommend bladder recurrence screening with cystoscopy should be performed with a frequency based upon the grade of the tumor, and follow the same guidelines as those for patients treated for bladder cancer. Upper tract imaging of the contralateral upper tract can be performed with retrograde ureteropyelography or CT urography at 1 year, then every 1–2 years.

Table 6.2 Technique of Surveillance Ureteroscopy

1. Cystourethroscopy
(a) Careful and complete
(b) 30° and 70° lens
2. Bladder lavage for cytology
3. Remove cystoscope
4. Rigid ureteroscopy
(a) Direct insertion of ureteroscope without a wire
(b) Leave wire through the ureteroscope to the level inspected
(c) Remove rigid ureteroscope, leaving guidewire in place
5. Flexible ureteroscopy
(a) Over the previously placed wire
(b) Inspect proximally from the level reached with rigid ureteroscope
6. Systematic inspection of intrarenal collecting system
(a) Fluoroscopy while irrigating with dilute contrast to ensure completeness
7. Aspirate intrarenal urine for cytology
8. Biopsy any suspicious lesions
9. Lavage for cytology after biopsy
10. Consider laser ablation of obvious urothelial carcinoma recurrence
11. Remove flexible ureteroscope and stent as indicated

The need for routine ureteroscopy outlined by these protocols has several potential disadvantages. One criticism has been the cost of frequent trips to the operating room compared to a single extirpative procedure. Endoscopic management is clearly more expensive than nephro-

Table 6.1 Summary of Surveillance Guidelines from the NCCN and EAU

	NCCN	EAU
Bladder		
Modality	Cystoscopy	Cystoscopy and cytology
Frequency	every 3 months for 1 year, then increasing intervals	at 3 months, 6 months, then every 6 months for 2 years, then annually
Upper tract		
Modality	IVP, CT urography, retrograde ureteropyelogram, ureteroscopy, or MRI urogram	Ureteroscopy
Frequency	3–12 months intervals	at 3 months, 6 months, then every 6 months for 2 years, then annually
Other	+/– CT, +/– CXR	CT urography at 3 months, 6 months then annually for at least 5 years

Fig. 6.2 Suggested surveillance protocol after endoscopic treatment of upper tract urothelial carcinoma

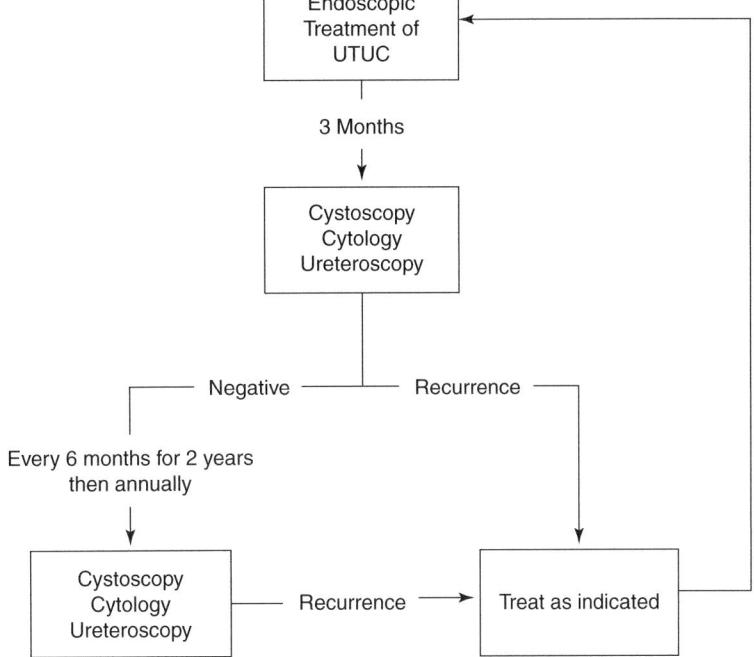

ureterectomy in patients who do not go on to develop chronic renal insufficiency following surgery. However, conservative management may be cost effective compared to nephroureterectomy and dialysis. One study found that performing endoscopic treatment of upper tract recurrences every 3 months for 5 years would still be $250,000 cheaper than undergoing nephroureterectomy and dialysis over the same time period [20].

Independent of cost, surveillance ureteroscopy under anesthesia carries with it inherent risks and is inconvenient for patients. In an effort to overcome the limitations of intensive ureteroscopic surveillance, office-based cystoureteroscopy techniques have been reported [14, 22]. Office-based ureteroscopy is facilitated by unroofing the ipsilateral ureteral orifice in the operating room at the time of initial surveillance ureteroscopy if no recurrence is detected [22]. Subsequent surveillance procedures can usually be performed in the office with minimal discomfort and risk to the patient. One study found a cost savings of $2912 per office-based surveillance procedure [14].

6.4   Surveillance Ureteroscopy Technique

The primary goal of surveillance or diagnostic ureteroscopy is an unhindered visual inspection of the entire upper urinary tract. There are some technical nuances that will help achieve this goal that will be discussed below.

Authors have reported performing flexible ureteroscopy without any guidewires (working or a safety). Some flexible ureteroscopes can be introduced into the ureteral orifice under direct vision without the use of a working guidewire [13]. Although this technique may become the ideal "no touch" method for diagnostic ureteroscopy, and will likely be technically easier with future generations of ureteroscopes, it is currently limited to certain ureteroscopes in the hands of experienced endourologists. For these reasons, we recommend and will review the standard technique of diagnostic ureteroscopy using complementary rigid and flexible ureteroscopy to inspect the entire upper urinary tract.

Surveillance endoscopy begins with thorough cystourethroscopy. This includes complete inspection of all segments of the urethra, a site of possible urothelial carcinoma recurrence. The bladder urothelium is then carefully and completely inspected and a bladder lavage for cytology is performed.

Rigid and flexible ureteroscopy provide complimentary access to the upper urinary tract [1]. Rigid ureteroscopy allows direct insertion and easy control of the ureteroscope, but access to the ureter superior to the iliac vessels is difficult and often not safely possible. Without active deflection of the ureteroscope tip, inspection of the intrarenal collecting system is impossible with a rigid ureteroscope. Flexible ureteroscopy provides complete access of the entire intrarenal collecting system and upper ureter. However, inspection of the distal ureter is difficult because of buckling of the ureteroscope into the bladder. For this reason, rigid ureteroscopy is performed below the iliac vessels, and flexible ureteroscopy above. This combination of rigid and flexible ureteroscopy provides safe, complete visual inspection of the entire upper urinary tract.

Conventional ureteroscopy technique can produce traumatic lesions that while innocuous, may be mistaken for pathology when performing ureteroscopy for tumor surveillance, or other diagnostic purposes. Therefore, care must be taken to minimize trauma to the ureter, as it will interfere with diagnostic visual inspection. The effort to minimize trauma begins with using the smallest ureteroscope practical to avoid the need for dilation. Direct insertion of a rigid ureteroscope without prior dilation of the intramural ureter allows clean inspection of the distal ureteral mucosa. Avoiding the use of a guide wire during direct insertion of the rigid ureteroscope will further minimize trauma to the ureter. The ureter is inspected with the rigid ureteroscope from the ureteral orifice to the ureter at the level of the iliac vessels. Avoidance of the use of ureteral access sheaths is advised to decrease ureteral trauma, and is seldom necessary for diagnostic ureteroscopy. Just enough irrigation is used to provide adequate distention of the ureter for visualization while preventing over distention of the ureter and intrarenal collecting system. Even minimal over-distention of the collecting

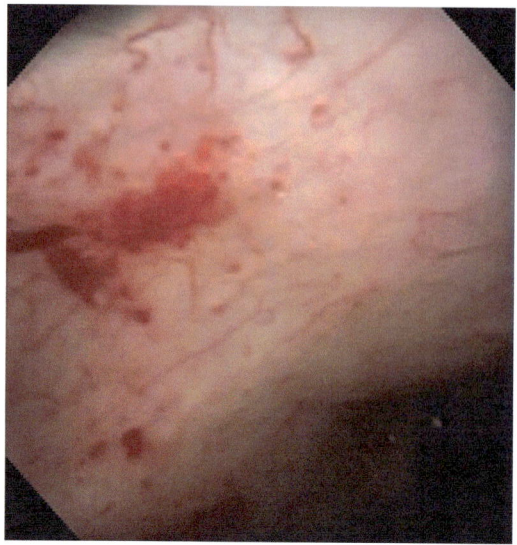

Fig. 6.3 Small areas of trauma from over-distention of the collecting system. Although of no direct clinical consequence, these areas can obscure ureteroscopic tumor detection, and should be avoided

system can lead to small areas of urothelial trauma that can be confused with tumor (Fig. 6.3).

Once the distal ureter is completely inspected to the level of the iliac vessels, further inspection of the proximal ureter requires flexible ureteroscopy. A guide wire is passed through the rigid ureteroscope, just far enough into the ureter to allow placement of the flexible ureteroscope. Preferably, the guide wire is passed only to the level of the ureter that had been inspected with the rigid ureteroscope. The rigid ureteroscope is removed, leaving the guide wire in place, and the flexible ureteroscope is passed over the wire to the proximal extent of rigid ureteroscopic inspection. Flexible ureteroscopy is performed proximally from this point, in a retrograde fashion, without a safety guide wire. Again, this is to avoid trauma to the ureteral urothelium that might interfere with diagnostic inspection.

When inspecting the intrarenal collecting system, completeness is ensured through a systematic approach using combined endoscopic and fluoroscopic imaging. Irrigation with a dilute contrast fluid mixed in normal saline allows precise documentation and navigation throughout the intrarenal collecting system. The intrarenal collecting system is inspected from the upper pole moving systematically through the calyces to the lower pole. Each calyx inspected is documented fluoroscopically. Care must be taken to minimize urothelial trauma by avoiding over-distention of the intrarenal collecting system. A nontraumatic approach to diagnostic ureteroscopy is essential.

Ureteroscopy is truly an endoscopic extension of cystoscopic principles to the upper urinary tract. Ureteroscopic inspection of the upper urinary tract allows direct visualization and recognition of pathologic lesions, just as during cystoscopy. Visual inspection of the upper urinary tract permits visual recognition and differentiation of upper urinary tract pathology. Transitional cell carcinoma generally has a distinctive appearance. However, some lesions, such as high-grade transitional cell carcinoma, may be difficult to distinguish from benign soft-tissue lesions such as inflammation. Ureteroscopic sampling for cytologic and pathologic analysis greatly improves our ability to distinguish malignant from benign soft-tissue lesions. Direct irrigation through the ureteroscope with normal saline and aspiration for cytology is done whenever there is the possibility of a malignant lesion. Biopsy performed under ureteroscopic visualization permits a more accurate diagnosis than brush biopsy of a lesion guided by fluoroscopy alone.

Biopsy of suspicious lesions can be performed with 3 French biopsy forceps for sessile lesions, or flat wire baskets for papillary lesions [15]. These samples can be preserved in formalin, and sent to pathology. Smaller samples should be preserved appropriately and examined using cytopathology techniques. Normal saline irrigated and aspirated through the working channel of the ureteroscope adjacent to the lesion can be sent to cytology as a wash specimen. Tumors can be treated ureteroscopically with the holmium laser, electrocautery, and/or the neodymium: YAG (Nd:YAG) laser, and these techniques are discussed in other chapters.

Conclusion

Improvements in the techniques and instrumentation of ureteroscopy have dramatically improved our ability to evaluate and treat patients with upper urinary tract urothelial carcinoma. Increasingly, patients are being treated in a minimally invasive fashion. These patients have a high rate of recurrence, so safe, thorough surveillance is critical to the detection of recurrences and appropriate treatment. The diagnostic ureteroscopy techniques described in this chapter can help us achieve this goal. The future of diagnostic ureteroscopy is bright, and will likely continue to expand as ureteroscopes, tissue sampling methods, and methods of intervention incrementally improve. Further research is needed to help define the most appropriate surveillance protocols and treatment options for patients with the often challenging problem of upper tract urothelial carcinoma.

Literature Cited

1. Bagley DH, Huffman JL, Lyon ES. Combined rigid and flexible ureteropyeloscopy. J Urol. 1983; 130:243–4.
2. Bagley DH, Rivas D. Thomas Jefferson University Philadelphia Pennsylvania. Department of Urology. Upper urinary tract filling defects: flexible ureteroscopic diagnosis. J Urol. 1990;143:1196–200.
3. Bagley DH. Ureteroscopic laser treatment of upper urinary tract tumors. J Clin Laser Med Surg. 1998; 16:55–9.
4. Chen GL, El-Gabry EA, Bagley DH. Surveillance of upper urinary tract transitional cell carcinoma: the role of ureteroscopy, retrograde pyelography, cytology and urinalysis. J Urol. 2000;164:1901–4.
5. Cutress ML, Stewart GD, Zakikhani P, Phipps S, Thomas BG, Tolley DA. Ureteroscopic and percutaneous management of upper tract urothelial carcinoma: systematic review. BJU Int. 2012;110: 614–28.
6. David KA, Mallin K, Milowsky MI, Ritchey J, Carroll PR, Nanus DM. Surveillance of urothelial carcinoma: stage and grade migration, 1993-2005 and survival trends, 1993-2000. Cancer. 2009;115:1435–47.
7. Elliott DS, Blute ML, Patterson DE, Bergstralh EJ, Segura JW; Mayo Clinic Department of Urology; Minnesota 55905 USA. Mayo Foundation. Long-term follow-up of endoscopically treated upper urinary tract transitional cell carcinoma. Urology. 1996; 47:819–25.
8. Go AS, Chertow GM, Fan D, McCulloch CE, HSU C. Chronic kidney disease and the risks of death, cardiovascular events, and hospitalization. NEJM. 2004;351:1296–305.

9. Grasso M, Fraiman M, Levine M; New York USA. Department of Urology. Ureteropyeloscopic diagnosis and treatment of upper urinary tract urothelial malignancies. Urology. 1999;54:240–6.

10. Grasso M, Fishman AI, Cohen J, Alexander B; Valhalla New York USA. Department of Urology. Ureteroscopic and extirpative treatment of upper urinary tract urothelial carcinoma: a 15-year comprehensive review of 160 consecutive patients. BJU Int. 2012;110:1618–26.

11. Hudson RG, Conlin MJ, Bagley DH; Division of Urology; Portland OR 97201-3098 USA. Renal Transplantation. Ureteric access with flexible ureteroscopes: effect of the size of the ureteroscope. BJU Int. 2005;95:1043–4.

12. Jemal A, Tiwari RC, Murray T, Ghafoor A, Samuels A, Ward E, Feuer EJ, Thun MJ. Cancer statistics, 2004. CA Cancer J Clin. 2004;54:8–29.

13. Johnson GB, Portela D, Grasso M; New York Medical College New York New York USA. Department of Urology. Advanced ureteroscopy: wireless and sheathless. J Endourol. 2006;20:552–5.

14. Jones SJ, Streem SB. Office-based cystoureteroscopy for assessment of the upper urinary tract. J Endourol. 2002;16:307–9.

15. Keeley FX, Kulp DA, Bibbo M, McCue PA, Bagley DH; Philadelphia Pennsylvania USA. Department of Urology. Diagnostic accuracy of ureteroscopic biopsy in upper tract transitional cell carcinoma. J Urol. 1997;157:33–7.

16. Luo HL, Kang CH, Chen YT, Chuang YC, Lee WC, Cheng YT, et al. Diagnostic ureteroscopy independently correlates with intravesical recurrence after nephroureterectomy for upper urinary tract urothelial carcinoma. Ann Surg Oncol. 2013;20:3121–6.

17. Martínez-Piñeiro JA, García Matres MJ, Martínez-Piñeiro L; Faculty of Medicine Universidad Autónoma Madrid Spain. Urological Service. Endourological treatment of upper tract urothelial carcinomas: analysis of a series of 59 tumors. J Urol. 1996;156:377–85.

18. National Kidney and Urological Diseases Information Clearinghouse, National Institute of Diabetes and Digestive and Kidney Disease (NIDDK). National Institutes of Health. NIH Publication 04-3895, 2004.

19. Munoz JJ, Ellison LM. Upper tract urothelial neoplasms: incidence and survival during the last 2 decades. J Urol. 2000;164:1523–5.

20. Pak RW, Moskowitz EJ, Bagley DH. What is the cost of maintaining a kidney in upper-tract transitional-cell carcinoma? An objective analysis of cost and survival. J Endourol. 2009;23:341–6.

21. Razdan S, Johannes J, Cox M, Bagley DH. Current practice patterns in urologic management of upper-tract transitional-cell carcinoma. J Endourol. 2005;19:366–71.

22. Reisiger K, Hruby G, Clayman RV, Landman J. Office-based surveillance ureteroscopy after endoscopic treatment of transitional cell carcinoma: technique and clinical outcome. Urology. 2007;70:263–6.

23. Rouprêt M, Babjuk M, Comp´erat E, Zigeuner R, Sylvester R, Burger M, et al. European guidelines on upper tract urothelial carcinomas: 2013 update. Eur Urol. 2013;63:1059–71.

24. Sagalowsky AI, Jarrett TW, Flanigan RC. Urothelial tumors of the upper urinary tract and ureter. In: Campbell-Walsh urology. 10th ed. Philadelphia: WB Saunders; 2011. p. 1516–53.

25. Stoller ML, Gentle DL, McDonald MW, Reese JH, Tacker JR, Carroll PR, et al. Endoscopic management of upper tract urothelial tumors. Tech Urol. 1997;3:152–7.

26. Tawfiek E, Bibbo M, Bagley DH. Ureteroscopic biopsy: technique and specimen preparation. Urology. 1997;50:117–9.

Topical Chemotherapy

7

John Michael Henderson and Francis X. Keeley Jr.

7.1 Introduction

The gold-standard treatment of upper tract urothelial carcinoma (UTUC) is radical nephroureterectomy. The benefits of oncological control must be carefully balanced against the loss of a renal unit, particularly in those patients with an anatomically or functionally solitary kidney, bilateral disease or chronic renal failure. The aim of topical treatment is to preserve the renal unit while maintaining acceptable oncological control.

The use of intravesical chemotherapy is well established in treating tumours of the lower urinary tract. There has been considerable interest in treating upper tract tumours in the same manner as they share the same urothelial surface.

7.2 Delivery Techniques

The constant flow of urine in the upper tract and lack of a storage organ such as the bladder presents a challenge of ensuring adequate urothelial exposure to the chosen agent. The three main delivery methods include;

1. antegrade via a nephrostomy catheter
2. retrograde via a ureteral catheter
3. allowing vesico-ureteral reflux via a double-pigtail stent.

The agents can be given as a continuous infusion or in boluses. The continuous infusion has the advantage of allowing for pressure monitoring, but may not allow for adequate exposure of the intrarenal collecting system as the agent may be carried away in the urine. It is imperative with all three methods that a low infusion pressure is used to prevent pyelolymphatic and pyelovenous backflow. When instilling the solution in a bolus, one must also keep in mind the capacity of the upper urinary tract, which is limited in most patients to 10–15 ml. A variation of the retrograde ureteral catheter is that of Patel and Fuchs where the ureteral catheter is brought out to the skin via the suprapubic route [1].

In an ex-vivo porcine model, Pollard et al. measured the percentage of upper tract urothelium stained by continuous infusion over 1 h of indigo carmine solution via the three methods [2]. An open ended ureteral catheter resulted in 83.6 % of surface area stained versus 65.2 and 66.2 % for the nephrostomy and refluxing double-pigtail stent respectively.

A course of treatment is required with BCG, which requires either a long-term nephrostomy, repeated insertion of a retrograde catheter, or the

J.M. Henderson, BMBS, BMedSci(Hons), FRCS, FEBU (✉) • F.X. Keeley Jr., MD, FRCS (Urol)
Bristol Urological Institute, Southmead Hospital, Bristol, UK
e-mail: john_henderson@doctors.net.uk; fxkeeley@gmail.com

© Springer International Publishing Switzerland 2015
M. Grasso III, D.H. Bagley (eds.), *Upper Urinary Tract Urothelial Carcinoma*,
DOI 10.1007/978-3-319-13869-5_7

technique described by Patel and Fuchs above; by contrast, mitomycin in typically given as a single dose with a ureteral catheter.

7.3 BCG Treatment

Bacillus Calmette- Guérin (BCG) is attenuated mycobacterium which demonstrates an immuno-modulatory effect which treats urothelial cancer.

It plays an important role in reducing the recurrence and progression rate of non-muscle invasive bladder cancer [3]. It is used in the upper tract as a potentially curative treatment in CIS or adjuvant treatment after endoscopic management of TCC.

The use of BCG to treat CIS of the upper tract has been described in a number of small retrospective series (Table 7.1). All series describe a 6-week course of weekly instillations with the

Table 7.1 Results of topical BCG for primary CIS

Group (year)	Patients (renal units)	Route	Initial positive response	Recurrence	Follow up (months)	Side effects/ complications
Studer [14] (1989)	8 (10)	Antegrade	4/8 (50 %)	2/8 (25 %)	18–28	Life-threatening septicaemia (1)
Sharpe [15] (1993)	11 (17)	Retrograde	8/11 (73 %)	2/11 (18 %)	11–64	Fever requiring antituberculous therapy (1) Haematuria (3)
Yokogi [16] (1996)	5 (8)	Antegrade (5) Retrograde (3)	5/8 (63 %)	0/8 (0 %)	10–46	Ureteric stricture (1) Renal tuberculosis (1) High fever (2)
Nonomura [17] (2000)	11 (11)	Retrograde	9/11 (82 %)	2/9 (22 %)	Not reported	Bladder irritability (8) Fever >38° (4) Haematuria (2)
Okubo [18] (2001)	11 (14)	Antegrade (2) Retrograde (12)	9/14 (64 %)	5/11 (45 %)	18–82	Not reported
Irie [19] (2002)	9 (13)	Retrograde	9/9 (100 %)	1/9 (11 %)	8–97	Irritable bladder (5) Fever >38.5° (2) Haematuria (2) Arthritis (1)
Thalman [9] (2002)	22 (25)	Antegrade	22/25 (88 %)	13/25 (52 %)	8–137	Fever, flu-like symptoms, LUTS (84 %) Fever >38° (4) Severe septicaemia (1) Fatal septicaemia (1)
Miyake [20] (2002)	16	Antegrade (5) Retrograde (11)	13/16 (81 %)	3/16 (19 %)	9–90	Bladder irritability (12) Fever >38° (9)
Hayashida [5] (2004)	10 (11)	Antegrade (4) Retrograde (6)	11/11 (100 %)	5/10 (50 %)	50.9	Bladder irritation (10) Fever >38° (9) Haematuria (2) Ureteral stenosis (1) Lumbago (1)
Kojima [4] (2006)	11 (13)	Retrograde	10/13 (77 %)	2/11 (8 %)	1–120	Fatal interstitial pneumonia (1)
Giannarini [10] (2011)	(42)	Antegrade	Not reported	17/42 (40 %)	42	Fever (5) Storage LUTS (5) Pericarditis (1) Infection/septicaemia (3) Fatal E. Coli septicaemia (1)

exception of Kojima et al. who gave an 8 week course [4]. The change of urine cytology from positive to negative is the usual criterion used to define response and a rate of greater than 60 % is reported. Further treatment was usually given if cytology remained positive. A subsequent recurrence rate of up to 55 % is described. Hayashida et al. found a recurrence rate of 50 % with mortality in all patients with recurrence [5]. They then introduced a more stringent radiological and endoscopic surveillance regimen which resulted in a significantly decreased recurrence rate. The use of cytology alone is now generally considered inadequate for surveillance, which raises questions about the actual efficacy reported in these small case series.

BCG is also used an adjuvant treatment after endoscopic treatment of UTUC. The series describing this treatment are shown in Table 7.2. A wide variation in recurrence rates are shown. Rastinehad et al noted no significant difference in time to recurrence, recurrence or progression rates between those groups treated with adjuvant BCG versus those who had no treatment [6]. It is important to note that all of these are retrospective, non-randomised studies.

7.3.1 Complications and Side Effects

A fever is a common finding during UTUC treatment with BCG. Schnapp et al found no clear association with symptoms, renal pelvic pressure or pre-treatment biochemical parameters in a series of patients treated though a nephrostomy, one of whom died of overwhelming sepsis [7]. They found that sepsis was more likely to be caused by typical uropathogens rather than BCG, presumably due to the colonization of a long-term nephrostomy.

Asymptomatic granulomatous involvement of the renal pelvis was found in 25 % of patients biopsied although the significance of this is unclear [8]. Hayashida et al introduced prophylactic isoniazid treatment halfway through their series to counter this risk [5]. Ureteral stenosis and hydronephrosis were noted in two patients in this same series although this could not conclusively be attributed to BCG. We have noted granulomas in the ureter causing strictures that preclude endoscopic surveillance, resulting in nephroureterectomy.

Fatal overwhelming sepsis is a rare but consistently reported complication in a number of series [4, 7, 9, 10].

Table 7.2 Results of upper tract BCG as adjuvant treatment after endoscopic treatment

Group (year)	Patients (renal units)	Route	Recurrence	Follow up (months)	Side effects/complications
Schoenberg [21] (1991)	9 (9)	Antegrade (4) Retrograde (5)	3/9 (33 %)	24	Fever and haematuria (1)
Vasavada [22] (1995)	8 (8)	Antegrade	1/8 (13 %)	22	Renal insufficiency (1)
Patel [1] (1998)	13 (17)	Retrograde	2/17 (12 %)	15	Candida albicans UTI (1) Persistent fevers (1)
Clark [23] (1999)	17 (18)	Antegrade	6/18 (33 %)	21	Not reported
Thalman [9] (2002)	15 (16)	Antegrade	14/16 (87 %)	42	Fever, flu-like symptoms, LUTS (84 %) Fever >38° (4) Severe septicaemia (1) Fatal septicaemia (1)
Rastinehad [6] (2009)	(50)	Antegrade	18/50 (36 %)	61	Fatal sepsis (1) Testicular granuloma requiring orchidectomy (1) BCG dissemination (1)
Giannarini [10] (2011)	(22)	Antegrade	13/22 (59 %)	42	Fever (5) Storage LUTS (5) Pericarditis (1) Infection/septicaemia (3) Fatal E. Coli septicaemia (1)

7.4   Mitomycin-C Treatment

Mitomycin-C (MMC) is an alkylating agent which is used to prevent recurrence of bladder TCC. It has been used in the adjuvant setting after endoscopic treatment of upper tract TCC at a dose of 40 mg. Martinez-Pineiro et al treated 14 renal units and demonstrated a recurrence rate of 14 % (2/14). Keeley and Bagley [11] treated 21 renal units with MMC after endoscopic treatment due to residual tumour (13), multifocal disease (10), higher grade tumour (3) or previous rapid recurrence after treatment (2). A complete response was seen in 45 % (9/19) and partial response in 37 % (7/19).

7.4.1   Complications and Side Effects

MMC is generally well tolerated. Fatal pneumonia due to agranulocytosis following mitomycin extravasation has been described [12] and reinforces the principle that a radiological imaging should be performed before infusion to exclude extravasation or obstruction. We restrict mitomycin instillation to a ureteral catheter rather than via a nephrostomy due to concerns about the risk of aplastic anemia. We have noted dense ureteral strictures on several occasions, resulting in nephroureterectomy due to the inability to survey the upper tract.

7.5   Other Treatments

Thiotepa is another alkylating agent which has been used to treat UTUC. Due to its low molecular weight, it may be systemically absorbed and cause haemopoietic toxicity. Martinez-Pineiro et al treated five patients with thiotepa and one with interferon-α2 [12]. The recurrence rate with thiotepa was 60 % compared to 12.5 % for BCG and 14.2 % although the absolute number of patients treated with thiotepa was small (n = 5).

In a series of 11 patients with upper tract CIS, Shapiro et al treated with a combination of BCG and interferon- α2B (50 million units) [13]. Their technique of delivery was via a ureteral catheter inserted under flexible cystoscopic guidance without the need for general anaesthesia. The patient group were candidates for both radical surgery and topical treatment. A more stringent follow up regimen included retrograde pyelography, flexible ureterenoscopy and rebiopsy of the upper tract. An initial complete response was seen in 73 % (8/11) with a further 2 patients completely responding after a second induction course. Patients who responded were placed on maintenance BCG therapy. The encouraging response rates were attributed to the addition of IFN to BCG, the use of maintenance BCG therapy, the novel delivery technique and the healthier patient group.

Conclusions

Topical chemotherapy may have a role to play in the treatment of UTUC, but the evidence supporting its use is weak. The use of BCG to treat primary CIS of the upper tract may be effective, but the reports to date include several that are based on negative urine cytology alone for surveillance. The subsequent recurrence rate of up to 50 % with a high mortality rate also raises some important issues. With the developments in urological technology, particular in respect to flexible ureterenoscopy, we believe that the regular use of ureteroscopy and biopsy should accompany the use of cytology for follow up. The side effects of fever and lower urinary tract symptoms are very common. In a small number of patients, treatment leads to overwhelming fatal infection and it is imperative to determine the risk factors that predispose to this. In the absence of clear efficacy, BCG should be used with caution. Likewise, the efficacy of mitomycin has not been proven but it appears to have a better safety profile.

The findings of these studies are limited by their small numbers of patients with heterogeneous disease (in terms of grade, multifocality and size), their retrospective nature and comparatively short follow up. There is a lack of consensus as to inclusion criteria, endoscopic, cytological and radiological follow up and definition of treatment success or failure.

A selection bias is inherent within most studies, with topical chemotherapy used for patients unfit for more radical surgery. Adequately-powered, randomised controlled trial could more accurately define the group who would most benefit from these treatments.

References

1. Patel A, Fuchs GJ. New techniques for the administration of topical adjuvant therapy after endoscopic ablation of upper urinary tract transitional cell carcinoma. J Urol. 1998;159(1):71–5.
2. Pollard ME, Levinson AW, Shapiro EY, Cha DY, Small AC, Mohamed NE, et al. Comparison of 3 upper tract anticarcinogenic agent delivery techniques in an ex vivo porcine model. Urology. 2013;82(6):1451. e1–6, Elsevier Inc.
3. Sylvester RJ, van der Meijden APM, Lamm DL. Intravesical bacillus Calmette-Guerin reduces the risk of progression in patients with superficial bladder cancer: a meta-analysis of the published results of randomized clinical trials. J Urol. 2002;168(5):1964–70.
4. Kojima Y, Tozawa K, Kawai N, Sasaki S, Hayashi Y, Kohri K. Long-term outcome of upper urinary tract carcinoma in situ: effectiveness of nephroureterectomy versus bacillus Calmette-Guérin therapy. Int J Urol. 2006;13(4):340–4.
5. Hayashida Y, Nomata K, Noguchi M, Eguchi J, Koga S, Yamashita S, et al. Long-term effects of bacille Calmette-Guérin perfusion therapy for treatment of transitional cell carcinoma in situ of upper urinary tract. Urology. 2004;63(6):1084–8.
6. Rastinehad AR, Ost MC, VanderBrink BA, Greenberg KL, El-Hakim A, Marcovich R, et al. A 20-year experience with percutaneous resection of upper tract transitional carcinoma: is there an oncologic benefit with adjuvant bacillus Calmette Guerin therapy? Urology. 2009;73(1):27–31.
7. Schnapp DS, Weiss GH, Smith AD. Fever following intracavitary bacillus Calmette-Guerin therapy for upper tract transitional cell carcinoma. J Urol. 1996;156(2 Pt 1):386–8.
8. Bellman GC, Sweetser P, Smith AD. Complications of intracavitary bacillus Calmette-Guerin after percutaneous resection of upper tract transitional cell carcinoma. J Urol. 1994;151(1):13–5.
9. Thalmann GN, Markwalder R, Walter B, Studer UE. Long-term experience with bacillus Calmette-Guerin therapy of upper urinary tract transitional cell carcinoma in patients not eligible for surgery. J Urol. 2002;168(4 Pt 1):1381–5.
10. Giannarini G, Kessler TM, Birkhäuser FD, Thalmann GN, Studer UE. Antegrade perfusion with bacillus Calmette-Guérin in patients with non-muscle-invasive urothelial carcinoma of the upper urinary tract: who may benefit? Eur Urol. 2011;60(5):955–60.
11. Keeley FX, Bagley DH. Adjuvant mitomycin C following endoscopic treatment of upper tract transitional cell carcinoma. J Urol. 1997;158(6):2074–7.
12. Martínez-Piñeiro JA, García Matres MJ, Martínez-Piñeiro L. Endourological treatment of upper tract urothelial carcinomas: analysis of a series of 59 tumors. J Urol. 1996;156:377–85.
13. Shapiro EY, Lipsky MJ, Cha DY, McKiernan JM, Benson MC, Gupta M. Outcomes of intrarenal Bacillus Calmette-Guérin/interferon-α2B for biopsy-proven upper-tract carcinoma in situ. J Endourol. 2012;26(12):1645–50.
14. Studer UE, Casanova G, Kraft R, Zingg EJ. Percutaneous bacillus Calmette-Guerin perfusion of the upper urinary tract for carcinoma in situ. J Urol. 1989;142:975–7.
15. Sharpe JR, Duffy G, Chin JL. Intrarenal bacillus Calmette-Guerin therapy for upper urinary tract carcinoma in situ. J Urol. 1993;149(3):457–9; discussion 459–60.
16. Yokogi H, Wada Y, Mizutani M, Igawa M, Ishibe T. Bacillus Calmette-Guérin perfusion therapy for carcinoma in situ of the upper urinary tract. Br J Urol. 1995;1996:676–9.
17. Nonomura N, Ono Y, Nozawa M, Fukui T, Harada Y, Nishimura K, et al. Bacillus Calmette-Guérin perfusion therapy for the treatment of transitional cell carcinoma in situ of the upper urinary tract. Eur Urol. 2000;38:701–4; discussion 705.
18. Okubo K, Ichioka K, Terada N, Matsuta Y, Yoshimura K, Arai Y. Intrarenal bacillus Calmette-Guerin therapy for carcinoma in situ of the upper urinary tract: Long-term follow-up and natural course in cases of failure. BJU Int. 2001;88(4):343–7.
19. Irie A, Iwamura M, Kadowaki K, Ohkawa A, Uchida T, Baba S. Intravesical instillation of bacille Calmette-Guerin for carcinoma in situ of the urothelium involving the upper urinary tract using vesicoureteral reflux created by a double-pigtail catheter. Urology. 2002;59(1):53–7.
20. Miyake H, Eto H, Hara S, Okada H, Kamidono S, Hara I. Clinical outcome of bacillus Calmette-Guerin perfusion therapy for carcinoma in situ of the upper urinary tract. Int J Urol. 2002;9(12):677–80.
21. Schoenberg MP, Van Arsdalen KN, Wein AJ. The management of transitional cell carcinoma in solitary renal units. J Urol. 1991;146(3):700–2; discussion 702–3.
22. Vasavada SE, Streem SB, Novick AC. Definitive tumor resection and percutaneous bacille Calmette-Guerin for management of renal pelvic transitional cell carcinoma in solitary kidneys. Urology. 1995;45(3):381–6.
23. Clark PE, Streem SB, Geisinger MA. 13-year experience with percutaneous management of upper tract transitional cell carcinoma. J Urol. 1999;161(3):772–6.

Systemic Chemotherapy for Upper Tract Urothelial Cancer

Jean Hoffman-Censits

8.1 Neoadjuvant Chemotherapy

8.1.1 Evidence Supporting Chemotherapy in Muscle Invasive Bladder Cancer

Though urothelial cancer is a common malignancy, particularly in older men, invasive high grade urothelial cancer of the upper tracts is a rare entity, for which there are no large prospective studies to guide care. Thus, chemotherapy in the perioperative setting for upper tract urothelial cancer is largely extrapolated from standard care for urothelial bladder cancer, which is more common. Level 1 evidence supports the use of standard mutli-day MVAC (methotrexate, vinblastine, adriamycin, cisplatin) chemotherapy prior to cystectomy for muscle invasive bladder cancer [5]. In the seminal prospective phase III study of MVAC prior to radical cystectomy (RC) compared to RC alone for patients with T2-T4a muscle invasive urothelial bladder cancer, patients the group who received MVAC had a significantly higher rate of pathologic complete response at RC than those in the RC alone arm (15 vs. 38 %). A statistically significant improvement in overall survival of 77 compared to 46 months with the addition of MVAC chemotherapy supports the use of this regimen for fit patients with muscle invasive urothelial bladder cancer prior to cystectomy ($p = 0.05$).

The toxicity of MVAC, and the relative comorbidity index of this population, who are typically older patients with smoking history, age related or renal comorbidities, has long precluded its widespread adoption. For patients with inoperable or metastatic urothelial bladder cancer, gemcitabine and cisplatin were prospectively compared to the multi-day MVAC regimen with comparable survival outcomes but with improved toxicity [26]. Based on these data and others, gemcitabine and cisplatin became the most commonly used regimen for bladder cancer in the community [1]. More recently, the EORTC performed a prospective phase III study of multi-day MVAC compared to accelerated or dose dense MVAC (DD-MVAC) in the advanced setting [24]. This regimen consists of the same doses of the MVAC regimen, but with all four agents given once every 14 days with myelocyte growth factor support. The dose dense regimen was better tolerated, and led to better outcomes. Recently 2 groups have published single arm prospective trials of DD-MVAC prior to cystectomy and have shown that it is a well-tolerated and efficient chemotherapy, and led to pathologic complete response outcomes similar to that reported with the less

J. Hoffman-Censits, MD
Department of Medical Oncology, Kimmel Cancer Center, Thomas Jefferson University Hospital, Philadelphia, PA 19107, USA
e-mail: Jean.Hoffman-Censits@jefferson.edu

© Springer International Publishing Switzerland 2015
M. Grasso III, D.H. Bagley (eds.), *Upper Urinary Tract Urothelial Carcinoma*,
DOI 10.1007/978-3-319-13869-5_8

well tolerated multi-day MVAC regimen [3, 16]. Large scale randomized studies have not been done, but based on these data and the EORTC study for patients with inoperable urothelial cancer, DD-MVAC has become the standard regimen used in the neoadjuvant and first line settings at many academic centers for patients with invasive bladder cancer.

8.1.2 Rationale for Neoadjuvant Chemotherapy for Upper Tract UC

Even with Level 1 evidence supporting traditionally dosed MVAC, the use of neoadjuvant chemotherapy for invasive urothelial bladder cancer remains a polarizing topic. Despite the data, some believe that only patients with high risk features, such as hydronephrosis and lymphovascular invasion, should get neoadjuvant treatment, or that adjuvant chemotherapy is as effective as neoadjuvant therapy. The dearth of prospective data for the use of chemotherapy in upper tract urothelial cancer can thus be even more polarizing. What is clear is that the opportunity to consider chemotherapy for patients with UTUC may be limited by a significant change in renal function postoperatively, which is required for the safe administration of cisplatin.

Aside from the potential improved tolerance of neoadjuvant chemotherapy, pathologic response at operative consolidation is a useful marker of chemosensitivity. In the original Grossman study of neoadjuvant MVAC, pathologic complete response (pCR) following TURBT alone or TURBT and MVAC chemotherapy appeared to correlate with improved survival [5]. Although pCR has not been prospectively validated to equate with overall survival, it is commonly used as a fast and reliable primary endpoint in neoadjuvant urothelial bladder studies. From the multi-institution Upper Tract Urothelial Cancer (UTUC) Collaboration of 12 international academic hospitals, survival updates from nine patients with pathologic complete response were reported [19]. Four of the nine

patients underwent neoadjuvant chemotherapy and lymphadenectomy while the remainder had endoscopic or no local therapy. Three patients developed recurrent disease, with a 5 year cancer specific survival estimate of 40 %.

8.1.3 Change in Renal Function Following Nephroureterectomy

As cisplatin is both metabolized by and is toxic to the kidney, safe administration of this agent is predicated upon reasonable renal function. Lane and colleagues reviewed 336 patients who had undergone nephroureterectomy (NU) at a single institution over 16 years [12]. They found a median 21 % loss of renal function following NU. This translated into a statistically significant increase in cisplatin ineligibility, based on generally accepted estimated glomerular filtration rate (GFR) of <60 mL/min/1.73 m^2, of 60 % ineligible prior to NU and 75 % ineligible following NU (p = 0.09). A similar retrospective study conducted in Asia found a 19.7 % decrease in GFR following nephroureterectomy, and not surprisingly, those over 65 years of age were the most vulnerable to this decline [20]. In a multi-institutional review of patients with UTUC and preoperative GFR >60, the median estimated GFR declined from 72 to 49 post nephroureterectomy and did not demonstrate recovery over time [9]. Patients who were older with lower preoperative GFR were the most vulnerable to decline in renal function postoperatively. A report of 666 patients who had undergone NU at seven international cancer centers showed a similar 18 % decline of renal function postoperatively [27]. The authors did not report an impact of GFR decline upon oncologic outcome, but only 9 % of patients in this series received neoadjuvant chemotherapy. In a Canadian multicenter series, GFR declined from a median of 59–47 following surgery, with only 19 % of patients with > pT3 or node positive disease able to receive some form of adjuvant therapy [28].

8.1.4 Evidence for Neoadjuvant Chemotherapy for Upper Tract UC

Data for the use of preoperative chemotherapy in upper tract urothelial cancer is predominantly retrospective. An early study from two Japanese centers evaluated 15 patients treated from 1988 to 1992 with three different methotrexate/cisplatin combinations, with two patients achieving a pathologic complete response [8]. In a single center retrospective series from MD Anderson, the impact of neoadjuvant chemotherapy on surgical outcomes following laparoscopic radical nephroureterectomy was evaluated [18]. Between 2003 and 2010, 82 patients underwent laparoscopic NU, 26 of whom received a median of 4 cycles of neoadjuvant chemotherapy, the majority of which was cisplatin based. Though there were no differences noted in surgical outcomes, there was a significant difference in rate of pathologic complete response, 15 % (4/26) in the patients who were offered preoperative chemotherapy compared to 1.7 % (1/56) for those who proceeded to surgery alone. The groups were relatively well balanced demographically and by other factors, though not surprisingly those who were offered preoperative chemotherapy had generally higher tumor grade than those who did not receive it.

In a single center retrospective series from MD Anderson of patients with high grade upper tract tumors, the outcomes of 43 patients treated with neoadjuvant chemotherapy followed by neprhoureterectomy between 2004 and 2008 were compared with 107 patients treated with nephroureterctomy alone between 1993 and 2004 [15]. Fourteen percent of patients who were treated with neoadjuvant chemotherapy achieved pathologic complete response, with comparable decrease in residual pT2 and T3 disease compared to the surgery alone group. The majority of patients received a cisplatin based combination therapy, with 44 % undergoing treatment with MVAC for a median of 4 cycles. An updated survival analysis from this dataset, evaluating only those patients with clinically node negative disease and high grade pathology by biopsy, was performed [17]. For this dataset, 24.7 % of patients who underwent up front nephroureterectomy had adjuvant chemotherapy, whereas none of the patients who had neoadjuvant chemotherapy did. Between the groups, there was a significant difference in rates of regional lymphadenectomy, reflecting change in surgical standards in the modern neoadjuvant group. The 5 year rate of overall survival was significantly higher in the patients who underwent neoadjuvant chemotherapy compared to those who did not, (80.2 % vs. 57.6 %, p=0.02).

The use of preoperative chemotherapy for clinically lymph node positive patients with UTUC, defined as >10 mm in short axis, was evaluated retrospectively at a single Japanese center [11]. Between 1995 and 2010 a total of 195 patients underwent an NU for UTUC, 29 of whom had radiographic evidence of loco regional lymphadenopathy. Fifteen of the 29 patients underwent neoadjuvant chemotherapy with either 2 or 3 cycles of MVAC or gemcitabine and cisplatin. No patient in this series had pathologic complete response, but 7 of the 15 who underwent neoadjuvant chemotherapy had down staging from initial clinical assessment, while none of the patients who underwent surgery alone had tumor down staging. There was an improvement in overall survival in the patients who underwent preoperative chemotherapy compared to those who did not (38 vs. 9 months), and a significant difference in survival in those patients who achieved pathologic down staging with chemotherapy compared to those who did not (3 year overall survival 83 vs. 33 %, p=0.041).

Two prospective studies of dose intensified neoadjuvant MVAC therapy in UTUC have been presented in abstract form. Sixteen patients with high grade upper tract tumors were included in a prospective study of neoadjuvant dose intensified MVAC with bevacizumab, in which 38 % of patients with upper tract tumors had pathologic complete response [22]. In a multi-institution prospective study of ten patients undergoing neoadjuvant MVAC, one attained pathologic complete response [7]. In both studies chemotherapy was well tolerated with expected toxicity, and no treatment related deaths. In these and the above retrospective series, rates of pCR tend be lower in upper tract malignancies compared to most reports in bladder cancer following neoadjuvant chemotherapy. This is likely due to aggressive transurethral resection of bladder tumor (TURBT) in addition to chemotherapy for bladder cancer, which is more difficult to achieve endoscopically for ureteral and renal pelvis cancers.

8.2 Adjuvant Chemotherapy

8.2.1 Evidence for Adjuvant Chemotherapy for Upper Tract UC

There are significantly more published retrospective series on the use of adjuvant chemotherapy following nephroureterectomy for upper tract urothelial cancer than neoadjuvant experiences. Mixed populations of patient pathologic tumor stage, retrospective data collection, use of either heterogeneous chemotherapy regimens or no report of the type of regimen used, make interpretation of these reports challenging.

Three retrospective series targeted patients with pT2 or T3 node negative disease following nephroureterectomy. In a small single center Korean study, 27 patients with pT3N0M0 upper tract tumors were evaluated, 16 of whom received adjuvant MVAC chemotherapy after all were approached for chemotherapy consideration [13]. The authors reported no difference in recurrence free or overall survival in this series based on receipt of chemotherapy. From a single Japanese institution, charts of 46 patients with pT2 or T3 node negative tumors were reviewed [23]. Between 1 and 3 cycles of MVAC were given to 24 of the 46 patients, offered only to those <80 years of age and with GFR >60. Though there was no difference in rates of 10 year overall survival (87.8 % for those who received adjuvant chemotherapy compared to 86.5 % for those that did not), there was a significantly higher rate of bladder cancer and systemic recurrence in those not offered adjuvant chemotherapy. In a multicenter Japanese report, 93 patients with pT3N0 urothelial cancer underwent a median of 2 cycles

of predominantly MVAC or other cisplatin combination chemotherapy [10]. Patients who received adjuvant chemotherapy were reported to have higher rates of 5 year relapse free and cancer specific survival than those who did not receive adjuvant chemotherapy, (CSS adjuvant 80.8 % compared to 64.4 % no chemotherapy). There was one chemotherapy associated death in this study due to myelosuppresion.

Several large studies evaluating adjuvant chemotherapy in mixed populations of patients with tumor stage >pT2 with or without lymph node positivity have been published. The largest series was from the 2009 report of the adjuvant chemotherapy experience from the international Upper Tract Urothelial Carcinoma Collaboration comprising 1390 patients. In this report, 542 high risk patients, defined as pT3 or pT4 and or lymph node positive, were evaluated [6]. Of these, 22 % underwent adjuvant chemotherapy, the majority of which was cisplatin based. Patients who received adjuvant chemotherapy tended to be younger with better functional status and high grade tumors, though the authors did not define criteria for offering adjuvant chemotherapy. They concluded that receipt of adjuvant chemotherapy did not impact on survival. In a similar high risk population identified from another multicenter cohort, of 627 patients with pT3 or pT4 or node positive UTUC, as well as 31 patients with distant metastasis, 22.6 % underwent predominantly platinum based regimens, offered based on fitness and adequacy of renal function [25]. Again adjuvant therapy did not confer a benefit in overall survival, but more patients offered adjuvant chemotherapy had positive lymph nodes or distant metastasis, indicative of a likely biased higher risk population than those not offered chemotherapy. Finally in a recently published Japanese multicenter experience, of 839 patients who had undergone nephroureterectomy, 229 had a high risk feature of pT3 or 4, tumor grade 3, lymphovascular invasion or lymph node involvement [21]. Eighty five of the 229 patients underwent chemotherapy, predominantly with MVAC or cisplatin and gemcitabine. Reasons for offering chemotherapy, and which regimen, were not reviewed, and the median numbers of cycles of

2.4 for MVAC and 2.2 for GC were similar. Overall the receipt of adjuvant chemotherapy did not appear to impact cancer specific survival, however evaluation of just those 85 patients who underwent chemotherapy suggested that the cancer specific survival was significantly higher for those who were treated with MVAC compared to gemcitabine and cisplatin.

Adjuvant chemotherapy use was evaluated in one series of 263 patients, all of whom had lymph node positive upper tract urothelial cancer, and thus a more homogenous population than in many series [14]. One of three cisplatin based regimens was given to 41 % of this population. Those who received adjuvant chemotherapy tended to be younger and with higher local stage and lymph node density. On multivariate analysis, use of adjuvant chemotherapy did not seem to affect rates of overall survival, but did improve relative mortality risk when only patients with pT3 and T4 tumors were included for analysis.

In one prospective published trial, 36 patients with pathologic T3 or 4 disease, or with any lymph node involvement following nephroureterectomy were included. Patients had to be without radiographic evidence of distant metastasis, and were enrolled to receive 4 cycles of carboplatin and paclitaxel to start between 4 and 6 weeks postoperatively [2]. Chemotherapy was exceptionally well tolerated, with 89 % of patients undergoing all cycles at full dose without delay, and with no treatment related deaths. The rate of 5 year overall survival was 52 %, and 17 of 36 patients developed local or metastatic relapse.

8.3   Cisplatin Eligibility

Cisplatin is the most active cytotoxic chemotherapy for urothelial cancers, but toxicities including mucositis, nausea and vomiting, ototoxicity, nephrotoxicity and neuropathy make it a challenging chemotherapy to tolerate. There are no concrete definitions for cisplatin eligibility; however, a consensus paper published by Galsky and colleagues provides guidance for medical oncologists [4]. In this publication, criteria used in prospective trials for "cisplatin unfit" patients with urothelial carcinoma, and survey data from genitourinary medical oncologists to define platinum eligibility, are summarized. Based on prior eligibility criteria in the reviewed trials, survey questions were generated, and a proposed consensus working group criteria for the cisplatin "unfit" was compiled. According to the authors, clinical trials designed to enroll patients who are cisplatin unfit could incorporate patients with one or more of the following comorbidities: Impaired functional status, impaired kidney function (creat clearance <60), impaired hearing, peripheral neuropathy, and impaired cardiac function. Importantly, the consensus for chemotherapy suitability was that renal function, regardless of nephrectomy status, should guide suitability for treatment.

Patients meeting one or more of these comorbid criteria meet eligibility requirements for clinical trials enrolling "cisplatin unfit" patients, though trial eligibility varies. Decision to deliver cisplatin based chemotherapy to patients with upper tract or bladder urothelial cancer outside of the clinical trial setting is at the discretion of the treating physician. This should happen with clear informed consent and discussion with the patient and caregivers regarding potential for toxicity, and strategies to manage and mitigate them.

Conclusion

High grade upper tract urothelial cancer is a disease associated with significant morbidity and mortality. As a rare entity, and with relatively few patients fit for cisplatin based regimens, prospective studies will continue to be lacking. Thus a clear understanding of the predominantly retrospective experience to date is crucial. Heterogeneity of chemotherapeutic regimens used in these studies, as well as patient baseline functional status and other medical comorbidities, tumor grade, stage and lymph node positivity, as well as variation in adequacy of lymphadenectomy, make interpretation of these retrospective studies even more challenging. For many adjuvant series, timing of chemotherapy postoperatively ranged from weeks to many months, and postoperative scans to rule out distant metastasis were not always done. Thus some of the poorer survival outcomes from adjuvant series may be reflective of patients treated in the first line for quickly recurrent disease post NU, rather than in the true adjuvant setting. What is clear is that following nephroureterectomy, GFR declines, which may preclude the delivery of effective chemotherapy. Multidisciplinary evaluations from urologic and medical oncology are imperative in this population as the opportunity for chemotherapy consideration may be lost in the postoperative setting, and informed consent given the lack of prospective data needs to be clear. In general, chemotherapy does appear to be beneficial in this population, and should be considered for those fit for cisplatin. Small prospective studies are ongoing. The first large scale prospective cooperative group trial, EA8141 A Phase II Trial of Neoadjuvant Systemic Chemotherapy Followed by Extirpative Surgery for Patients with High Grade Upper Tract Urothelial Carcinoma, has been recently activated. This study will provide information on tolerance and efficacy of neoadjuvant chemotherapy for this population.

References

1. Apolo AB, Kim JW, Bochner BH, Steinberg SM, Bajorin DF, Kevin Kelly W, Agarwal PK, Koppie TM, Kaag MG, Quinn DI, Vogelzang NJ, Sridhar SS. Examining the management of muscle-invasive bladder cancer by medical oncologists in the United States. Urol Oncol. 2014;32(5):637–44.
2. Bamias A, Deliveliotis C, Fountzilas G, Gika D, Anagnostopoulos A, Zorzou MP, Kastritis E, Constantinides C, Kosmidis P, Dimopoulos MA. Adjuvant chemotherapy with paclitaxel and carboplatin in patients with advanced carcinoma of the upper urinary tract: a study by the Hellenic Cooperative Oncology Group. J Clin Oncol. 2004;22(11):2150–4.
3. Choueiri TK, Jacobus S, Bellmunt J, Qu A, Appleman LJ, Tretter C, Bubley GJ, Stack EC, Signoretti S, Walsh M, Steele G, Hirsch M, Sweeney CJ, Taplin M, Kibel AS, Krajewski KM, Kantoff PW, Ross RW, Rosenberg JE. Neoadjuvant dose-dense Methotrexate, vinblastine, doxorubicin, and cisplatin with Pegfilgrastim support in muscle-invasive urothelial cancer: pathologic, radiologic, and biomarker correlates. J Clin Oncol. 2014;32(18):1889–94.
4. Galsky MD, Hahn NM, Rosenberg J, Sonpavde G, Hutson T, Oh WK, Dreicer R, Vogelzang N, Sternberg CN, Bajorin DF, Bellmunt J. Treatment of patients with metastatic urothelial cancer "unfit" for cisplatin-based chemotherapy. J Clin Oncol. 2011;29(17):2432–8.
5. Grossman HB, Natale RB, Tangen CM, Speights VO, Vogelzang NJ, Trump DL, White RWD, Sarosdy MF, Wood Jr DP, Raghavan D, Crawford ED. Neoadjuvant chemotherapy plus cystectomy compared with cystectomy alone for locally advanced bladder cancer. N Engl J Med. 2003;349(9):859–66.
6. Hellenthal NJ, Shariat SF, Margulis V, Karakiewicz PI, Roscigno M, Bolenz C, Remzi M, Weizer A, Zigeuner R, Bensalah K, Ng CK, Raman JD, Kikuchi E, Montorsi F, Oya M, Wood CG, Fernandez M, Evans CP, Koppie TM. Adjuvant chemotherapy for high risk upper tract urothelial carcinoma: results from the Upper Tract Urothelial Carcinoma Collaboration. J Urol. 2009;182(3):900–6.
7. Hoffman-Censits JH, Trabulsi EJ, Chen DYT, Kutikov A, Lin J, Viterbo R, Hudes GR, Healy KA, Hubosky S, Wong Y, Kilpatrick D, Adair B, Cione C, Plimack ER. Neoadjuvant accelerated methotrexate, vinblastine, doxorubicin, and cisplatin (AMVAC) in patients with high-grade upper-tract urothelial carcinoma. ASCO Meeting Abstr. 2014;32(4 Suppl):326.
8. Igawa M, Urakami S, Shiina H, Kishi H, Himeno Y, Ishibe T, Kadena H, Usui T. Neoadjuvant chemotherapy for locally advanced urothelial cancer of the upper urinary tract. Urol Int. 1995;55(2):74–7.
9. Kaag M, Trost L, Thompson RH, Favaretto R, Elliott V, Shariat SF, Maschino A, Vertosick E, Raman JD, Dalbagni G. Preoperative predictors of renal function decline after radical nephroureterectomy for upper tract urothelial carcinoma. BJU Int. 2014;114(5):674–9.
10. Kawashima A, Nakai Y, NAKAYAMA M, Ujike T, Tanigawa G, Ono Y, Kamoto A, TAKADA T, Yamaguchi Y, Takayama H, Nishimura K, Nonomura N, Tsujimura A. The result of adjuvant chemotherapy for localized pT3 upper urinary tract carcinoma in a multi-institutional study. World J Urol. 2012;30(5):701–6.
11. Kitamura H, Igarashi M, Tanaka T, Shindo T, Masumori N, Tamakawa M, Kawaai Y, Tsukamoto T. A role for preoperative systemic chemotherapy in node-positive upper tract urothelial carcinoma treated with radical nephroureterectomy. Jpn J Clin Oncol. 2012;42(12):1192–6.
12. Lane BR, Smith AK, Larson BT, Gong MC, Campbell SC, Raghavan D, Dreicer R, Hansel DE, Stephenson AJ. Chronic kidney disease after nephroureterectomy for upper tract urothelial carcinoma and implications for the administration of perioperative chemotherapy. Cancer. 2010;116(12):2967–73.
13. Lee SE, Byun SS, Park YH, Chang IH, Kim YJ, Hong SK. Adjuvant chemotherapy in the management of pT3N0M0 transitional cell carcinoma of the upper urinary tract. Urol Int. 2006;77(1):22–6.
14. Lucca I, Kassouf W, Kapoor A, Fairey A, Rendon RA, Izawa JI, Black PC, Fajkovic H, Seitz C, Remzi M, Nyirády P, Rouprêt M, Margulis V, Lotan Y, de Martino M, Hofbauer SL, Karakiewic PI, Briganti A, Novara G, Shariat SF, Klatte T. (2015), The role

of adjuvant chemotherapy for lymph node-positive upper tract urothelial carcinoma following radical nephroureterectomy: a retrospective study. BJU International. 2014;115:1–7 doi: 10.1111/bju.12801.

15. Matin SF, Margulis V, Kamat A, Wood CG, Grossman HB, Brown GA, Dinney CP, Millikan R, Siefker-Radtke AO. Incidence of downstaging and complete remission after neoadjuvant chemotherapy for high-risk upper tract transitional cell carcinoma. Cancer. 2010;116(13):3127–34.

16. Plimack ER, Hoffman-Censits JH, Viterbo R, Trabulsi EJ, Ross EA, Greenberg RE, Chen DYT, Lallas CD, Wong Y, Lin J, Kutikov A, DOTAN E, Brennan TA, Palma N, Dulaimi E, Mehrazin R, Boorjian SA, Kelly WK, Uzzo RG, Hudes GR. Accelerated methotrexate, vinblastine, doxorubicin, and cisplatin is safe, effective, and efficient neoadjuvant treatment for muscle-invasive bladder cancer: results of a multicenter phase II study with molecular correlates of response and toxicity. J Clin Oncol. 2014;32(18):1895–901.

17. Porten S, Siefker-Radtke AO, Xiao L, Margulis V, Kamat AM, Wood CG, Jonasch E, Dinney CP, Matin SF. Neoadjuvant chemotherapy improves survival of patients with upper tract urothelial carcinoma. Cancer. 2014;120(12):1794–9.

18. Rajput MZ, Kamat AM, Clavell-Hernandez J, Siefker-Radtke AO, Grossman HB, Dinney CP, Matin SF. Perioperative outcomes of laparoscopic radical nephroureterectomy and regional lymphadenectomy in patients with upper urinary tract urothelial carcinoma after neoadjuvant chemotherapy. Urology. 2011;78(1):61–7.

19. Raman JD, Ng CK, Shariat SF, Margulis V, Montorsi F, Karakiewicz P, Upper-Tract Urothelial Carcinoma Collaboration. Outcomes for patients with pT0 disease after radical nephroureterectomy for upper-tract urothelial carcinoma. BJU International. 2009;103(1):3–4.

20. Shao IH, Lin YH, Hou CP, Juang HH, Chen CL, Chang PL, Tsui KH. Risk factors associated with ineligibility of adjuvant cisplatin-based chemotherapy after nephroureterectomy. Drug Des Devel Ther. 2014;8:1985–90.

21. Shirotake S, Kikuchi E, Tanaka N, Matsumoto K, Miyazaki Y, Kobayashi H, Ide H, Obata J, Hoshino K, Kaneko G, Hagiwara M, Kosaka T, Kanao K, Kodaira K, Hara S, Oyama M, Momma T, Miyajima A, Nakagawa K, Hasegawa S, Nakajima Y, Oya M. Impact of an adjuvant chemotherapeutic regimen on the clinical outcome in high-risk patients with upper tract urothelial carcinoma: a Japanese multi-institution experience. J Urol. 2015;193(4):1122–8.

22. Siefker-Radtke AO, Kamat AM, Corn PG, Matin SF, Grossman HB, Millikan RE, Dinney CPN. Neoadjuvant chemotherapy with DD-MVAC and bevacizumab in high-risk urothelial cancer: results from a phase II trial at the M. D. Anderson Cancer Center. ASCO Meeting Abstr. 2012;30(5 Suppl):261.

23. Soga N, Arima K, Sugimura Y. Adjuvant methotrexate, vinblastine, adriamycin, and cisplatin chemotherapy has potential to prevent recurrence of bladder tumors after surgical removal of upper urinary tract transitional cell carcinoma. Int J Urol Off J Jpn Urol Assoc. 2008;15(9):800–3.

24. Sternberg CN, De Mulder PHM, Schornagel JH, Théodore C, Fossa SD, Van Oosterom AT, Witjes F, Spina M, Van Groeningen CJ, de Balincourt C, Collette L, For the European Organization for Research and Treatment of Cancer Genitourinary Tract Cancer Cooperative Group. Randomized phase III trial of high–dose-intensity Methotrexate, vinblastine, doxorubicin, and cisplatin (MVAC) chemotherapy and recombinant human granulocyte colony-stimulating factor versus classic MVAC in advanced urothelial tract tumors: European Organization for Research and Treatment of Cancer Protocol No. 30924. J Clin Oncol. 2001;19(10):2638–46.

25. Vassilakopoulou M, de la Motte Rouge T, Colin P, Ouzzane A, Khayat D, Dimopoulos MA, Papadimitriou CA, Bamias A, Pignot G, Nouhaud FX, Hurel S, Guy L, Bigot P, Roumiguie M, Roupret M, French Collaborative National Database on UUT-UCC. Outcomes after adjuvant chemotherapy in the treatment of high-risk urothelial carcinoma of the upper urinary tract (UUT-UC): results from a large multicenter collaborative study. Cancer. 2011;117(24):5500–8.

26. Von der Maase H, Hansen SW, Roberts JT, Dogliotti L, Oliver T, Moore MJ, Bodrogi I, Albers P, Knuth A, Lippert CM, Kerbrat P, Sanchez Rovira P, Wersall P, Cleall SP, Roychowdhury DF, Tomlin I, Visseren-Grul CM, Conte PF. Gemcitabine and cisplatin versus methotrexate, vinblastine, doxorubicin, and cisplatin in advanced or metastatic bladder cancer: results of a large, randomized, multinational, multicenter, phase III study. J Clin Oncol. 2000;18(17):3068–77.

27. Xylinas E, Rink M, Margulis V, Clozel T, Lee RK, Comploj E, Novara G, Raman JD, Lotan Y, Weizer A, Roupret M, Pycha A, Scherr DS, Seitz C, Ficarra V, Trinh QD, Karakiewicz PI, Montorsi F, Zerbib M, Shariat SF, UTUC Collaboration. Impact of renal function on eligibility for chemotherapy and survival in patients who have undergone radical nephro-ureterectomy. BJU International. 2013;112(4):453–61.

28. Yafi FA, Tanguay S, Rendon R, Jacobsen N, Fairey A, Izawa J, Kapoor A, Black P, Lacombe L, Chin J, So A, Lattouf J, Bell D, Fradet Y, Saad F, Matsumoto E, Drachenberg D, Cagiannos I, Kassouf W. Adjuvant chemotherapy for upper-tract urothelial carcinoma treated with nephroureterectomy: assessment of adequate renal function and influence on outcome. Urol Oncol Semin Orig Invest. 2014;32(1):31. e17–24.

Hereditary Upper Tract Urothelial Carcinoma: Lynch Syndrome, Hereditary Nonpolyposis Colorectal Cancer Syndrome (HNPCC)

9

Scott G. Hubosky and Bruce M. Boman

9.1 Introduction

Genetics and environment clearly both play a role in the pathogenesis of upper tract urothelial carcinoma (UTUC). This malignancy is heterogeneous in its phenotypical presentation among geographical locations in its sporadic forms, which both vary from it's hereditary form in Lynch Syndrome (LS), also known as hereditary nonpolyposis colorectal cancer (HNPCC) (Table 9.1). Lynch syndrome is among the most common Mendelian disorders and the population incidence of LS carriers is believed to be 1:370 in the United States [14]. This autosomal dominant cancer syndrome is characterized by germline mutations in DNA mismatch repair (MMR) genes, particularly *MSH-2*, *MLH-1*, *MSH-6* and *PMS-2*. Currently, it is estimated that LS is the responsible etiology for 2.4–3.7 % of all colorectal cancer (CRC) cases and 1.8–3.9 % of all endometrial cancer (EC) cases. The lifetime penetrance of LS genetic mutations for CRC is 25–70 % and for EC is 30–70 % [15]. Variation exists due to different penetrance rates for the possible MMR gene mutations for a given cancer type. UTUC as well as various other malignancies involving the small bowel, stomach, biliary tract, brain and skin (sebaceous neoplasms) have been shown to be part of the extra-colonic tumor spectrum in LS. LS trait carriers and patients with known *MSH-2* mutations have a relative risk of 75 for UTUC development compared to the general population [16]. In addition, our group and others have observed UTUC in families with *MSH-6* and *MLH-1* mutations albeit less often relative to those with alterations in *MSH-2*. Identification of these patients and affected family members is a high priority since they ultimately may benefit from early and frequent surveillance protocols.

9.2 Sporadic Forms of Upper Tract Urothelial Carcinoma: West Versus East

The epidemiology of sporadic cases of UTUC has been well defined in multiple reports over the years. As with other malignant tumors, age is a major risk factor. Typically UTUC is found in persons with median age 69–70 in large published series [1, 3–6]. Involvement of the renal pelvis has been reported to be two to four times more common compared to the ureter [1, 17]. Smoking is a well-defined risk factor and carries a three to

S.G. Hubosky, MD (✉)
Department of Urology, Thomas Jefferson
University, 1025 Walnut Street, Suite 1100,
Philadelphia, PA 19107, USA
e-mail: Scott.hubosky@jefferson.edu

B.M. Boman, MD, PhD
Department of Medical Oncology,
Thomas Jefferson University, 1025 Walnut Street,
Philadelphia, PA 19107, USA

© Springer International Publishing Switzerland 2015
M. Grasso III, D.H. Bagley (eds.), *Upper Urinary Tract Urothelial Carcinoma*,
DOI 10.1007/978-3-319-13869-5_9

Table 9.1 UTUC epidemiological characteristics vary with geography and genetic predisposition

Series	N	Country	Male/female ratio	Age on presentation
West				
Margulis et al. (2009) [1]	1,363	N. America West Europe	2.1/1	69.7
Audenet (2012) [44]	1,122	France	2.3/1	70.4
Shariat et al. (2011) [3]	785	N. America West Europe	2.2/1	68
Holmang and Johansson (2006) [4]	768	Sweden	1.4/1	67 (bilateral) 70 (unilateral)
Hall et al. (1998) [5]	252	USA	2.2/1	67 (women) 69 (men)
Grasso et al. (2012) [6]	160	USA	1.5/1	73
East				
Fang et al. (2014) [7]	892	China	0.8/1	67
Luo et al. (2013) [8]	396	Taiwan	0.9/1	66
Li et al. (2008) [9]	260	Taiwan	0.9/1	65
Milenkovic et al. (2014) [10]	203	Serbia	1.2/1	66
HNPCC				
Watson et al. (2008) [11]	82	USA Scandinavia West Europe	1.3/1	NA
Crokett et al. (2011) [12]	39	USA	0.95/1	62
Hubosky et al. (2013) [13]	13	USA	1.2/1	56

seven fold increased risk for UTUC development [18, 19]. Occupational exposure to hydrocarbons and/or petroleum products as seen by those working in the fields of chemistry, plastics, coal, tar and asphalt is thought to induce a relative risk of four to five for UTUC development [19]. Men are almost twice as likely than women to develop UTUC in most reports from western countries, similar to urothelial carcinoma of the bladder. In eastern countries plagued by Aristolochic acid nephropathy (AAN), also known as Balkan endemic nephropathy (BEN), there is a noted female predominance in large UTUC series [7–9] (Table 9.1). This trend is thought to be secondary to herbal use for weight-reduction [20] and the intermingling of *Aristolochia clematitis* seeds with wheat grain used to prepare home-baked bread in Balkan nations such as Croatia, Serbia, Romania, Bulgaria and Bosnia [21, 22]. Once thought to be familial in origin, BEN has since been traced to chronic exposure to herbs or seeds of all *Aristolochia* plants. Persons exposed to these nephrotoxic carcinogens tend to develop a progressive tubulointerstitial nephropathy culminating in UTUC in up to 50 % of cases [22].

9.3 HNPCC: Historical Perspective

In 1913, a published report by Dr. Aldred Warthin described a family in Michigan with multiple members suffering from colon and uterine cancers, which suggested an inheritance pattern [23]. Fifty years later, this expanded kindred was further studied by Dr. Henry Lynch and observations pointed to an autosomal dominant mode of inheritance of predominantly colorectal and endometrial carcinomas [24]. Clinical criteria, known as Amsterdam Criteria, focusing mostly on family history of colorectal cancer, emerged to better identify these individuals with HNPCC and to try to help standardize patient cohorts for study [25]. Later, human MMR genes were linked to cancer susceptibility in HNPCC families, further elucidating the molecular etiology of this cancer syndrome [26, 27]. In the early 1990s, UTUC was determined to be part of the tumor spectrum of hereditary nonpolyposis colorectal cancer (HNPCC) [28]. Given the new appreciation for extra-colonic tumors in the HNPCC spectrum, broader clinical criteria were proposed, known as Amsterdam Criteria II

Table 9.2 Amsterdam criteria II

Requires at least three relatives with an HNPCC associated cancer: (colorectal cancer; cancer of the endometrium, small intestine, ureter or renal pelvis; all of the following criteria should be present:
One should be a first degree relative of the other two;
At least two successive generations should be affected;
At least one should be diagnosed before age 50 years;
Familial adenomatous polyposis (FAP) should be ruled out in any present cases of colorectal cancer;
Tumors should be verified by pathologic examination.

Ref. [29], Reprinted with permission from Elsevier

(Table 9.2), which aimed to include not only patients with personal or family history of CRC, but also include those individuals with UTUC, endometrial carcinoma and small bowel malignancies [29]. The association of Microsatellite Instability (MSI) with tumors in HNPCC led to the incorporating of molecular testing of surgical specimen tissue in patients presenting with known HNPCC malignancies, especially CRC. The Bethesda Criteria were proposed to determine which patients with known HNPCC tumors would qualify for MSI testing, thus providing the potential for prospective molecular screening of HNPCC-related tumor tissue and enhancing the ability to identify LS carriers [30]. Today LS patients are usually first identified by either clinical history or prospective molecular screening of tumor tissue with MSI testing and immunohistochemistry (IHC) to detect the absence of proteins made by MMR genes *MSH-2, MLH-1, MSH-6* and *PMS-2*. In a patient meeting clinical criteria or with tumor tissues that are MSI high or demonstrating a missing MMR gene protein product on IHC, the diagnosis of LS is confirmed through germline genetic testing to detect the exact pathogenic mutation. Given the autosomal dominant inheritance pattern, family members can then be offered genetic testing to confirm or rule out their individual risk.

9.4   Incidence and Lifetime Risk of UTUC in LS Carriers

In 2008, members from four major LS research centers from the USA and Europe pooled their data to provide a retrospective cohort study in an effort to define the lifetime risk of developing extra-colonic and extra-endometrial cancers in LS patients and carriers [11]. This multi-institutional cohort consisted of over 6,000 individuals from 261 families with carrier or probable carrier status of a mutation in MSH-2 or MLH-1. Many first-degree relatives of these LS carriers were also included. The authors estimated an 8.4 % lifetime risk among LS carriers for the development of UTUC. Further risk stratification demonstrated the highest risk in men with MSH-2 mutations, assuming up to a 28 % lifetime UTUC risk. Women with MSH-2 mutations were noted to have a 12 % lifetime risk of UTUC development. The peak age for UTUC diagnosis was between ages 50 and 70. Prior to age 50, the risk of UTUC development was very low. There was a seven-fold higher risk for members of MSH-2 families versus those with MLH-1 mutations.

9.5   Characteristics of UTUC in Patients with Lynch Syndrome

Given the distinct historical behavior of CRC in LS compared to sporadic CRC, it is not surprising that LS patients with UTUC would have some diverse features from sporadic UTUC patients. The most common manifestation of LS is CRC and these cases have many interesting differences clinically and pathologically when compared to sporadic CRC cases. Patients with LS present with CRC at significantly younger ages compared to sporadic CRC cases (45 years versus 64 years, respectively) [31]. LS patients with CRC tend to have predominantly right-sided colon lesions, specifically proximal to the splenic flexure, and usually are more prone to multiple lesions presenting either simultaneously or over time [32]. Even though colon polyps are not necessarily more common in LS patients, polyps do occur at younger ages, tend to be larger in size, demonstrate more villous features and are more likely to contain contiguous adenocarcinoma when compared to patients with sporadic colon polyps [33]. Interestingly, multiple studies have shown that LS patients with CRC have a superior overall survival rate versus sporadic CRC cases when controlled for age and stage [34, 35]. Unfortunately, not as much information is yet available when comparing sporadic UTUC patients with those having UTUC and LS. This is mostly due to smaller numbers, lack of awareness and likely unrecognized cases.

The first descriptions of UTUC in Lynch syndrome came out of retrospective studies by medical oncology groups. Many factors make it difficult to draw any solid conclusions about the unique characteristics of UTUC in LS cases based on these early studies. These factors include how patient cohorts were picked for study inclusion, data organization and the limited amount of retrospective data available. Prior to the availability of genetic mutation analysis to provide for LS carrier designation, patient cohorts were initially identified by the use of Amsterdam Criteria I, which relies solely on the presence of family history of colon cancer [28, 36]. Not until the later introduction of Amsterdam Criteria II [29] and the Bethesda Criteria [37] did patients with extra-colonic malignancies get full consideration for inclusion. Therefore these early studies likely excluded some number of UTUC cases with LS. Additionally, the early cohort studies were sometimes lacking pathology report information and loosely characterized UTUC cases in the broad category of "GU malignancy" having them lumped together with urothelial carcinomas of the bladder or renal cell carcinomas. No mention was ever made about the presence or absence of synchronous or metachronous bilateral UTUC in these patients.

In order to highlight the characteristics of UTUC in LS, Crockett et al. presented a retrospective case-control study providing a formal comparison of UTUC in LS patients against a well-established cohort of sporadic UTUC cases from Sweden [12]. The LS patients were extracted from Creighton University's HNPCC database, which comprises a 42-year experience worth of data from patients with LS from 1964 to 2006. From the Creighton registry, a total of 39 patients were identified as having met Amsterdam Criteria II and having a diagnosis of UTUC. A total of 33/39 (85 %) of these patients had available genetic mutational analysis verifying MSH-2 or MLH-1 mutations and 26/39 (66 %) had formal pathological

grading and staging of their UTUC specimen on record. Thus, for a retrospective study, reasonably strict inclusion criteria for the LS cohort were met. For comparison, 783 patients from western Sweden with UTUC diagnosis served as the control group, representing sporadic cases. The two cohorts were statistically compared. Upon initial presentation, the LS/UTUC group was on average 8 years younger than the sporadic UTUC group (62 years and 70 years, respectfully). LS patients had a higher proportion of primary UTUC in the ureter (51 %) compared to the intrarenal collecting system (39 %). By contrast, sporadic UTUC patients had more intrarenal tumors (65 %) compared to ureteral lesions (28 %). Based on the 2004 WHO grading system for urothelial carcinoma, there were similar numbers of high-grade cases between LS and sporadic cases (88 % and 74 %, respectively). Interestingly, in the LS cohort, the male/female ratio was 0.95 while in the sporadic group it was 1.52. No statistically significant differences were noted in tumor staging or the subsequent development of de novo urothelial carcinomas of the bladder. Survival data and the presence of bilateral UTUC were not specifically addressed in this report. The authors noted that their study did not provide conclusive evidence to forgo nephroureterectomy (NU) for treatment of UTUC in LS, but nevertheless, they advised "considerable caution" should still be exercised prior to considering complete NU in these patients due to the potentially higher risk of later UTUC development in the contralateral renal unit.

Another retrospective study recently reported the effectiveness of ureteroscopic laser ablative treatment in LS patients with UTUC and also suggested the increased risk for bilateral upper tract disease in this unique population [13]. Thirteen patients were identified with UTUC and had documented MSH-2 mutations by germline mutation analysis. Similarly to the Crockett study, patients were relatively young at time of presentation with UTUC at mean age 56.5 years (range 38–73) and a greater tendency for ureteral tumor location was noted (66 %) compared to the intrarenal collecting system (33 %). Unlike Crockett's study, the majority of patients had low-grade disease (73 %) according to the 2004 WHO grading system for

Table 9.3 Upper tract urothelial carcinoma: sporadic vs HNPCC cases

Series	N	Age at presentation (years)	Incidence of bilateral UTUC (%)	Location: renal/ureteral/both
Sporadic cases				
Charbit et al. (1991) [38]	108	63.5	2.7 % (synchronous)	53 %/47 %
Holmang and Johansson (2006) [4]	781	67	3.1 %(metachronous) 1.6 % (synchronous)	65 %/28 %/7 %
Margulis et al. (2009) [1]	1,363	69.7	N/A	64 %/34 %
Fang et al. (2014) [7]	892	73	4.4 % (synchronous)	N/A
HNPCC cases				
Watson and Lynch (1993) [28]	12	56	N/A	58 %/42 %
Sijmons et al. (1998) [39]	7	58	N/A	N/A
Vasen et al. (1994) [36]	28	57	N/A	39 %/61 %
Crockett et al. (2011) [12]	39	62	0 %	39 %/51 %/8 %
Hubosky et al. (2013) [13]	13	56.5	46 % (metachronous) 0 % (synchronous)	33 %/67 %

urothelial carcinoma. When considering each patient's complete urological history, bilateral UTUC was noted in 6/13 (46 %). All six of these patients had metachronous disease presentation with a mean time of 49 months until bilateral UTUC development. The authors were careful to point out that selection bias obviously must be taken into consideration given that four of the six patients had extirpative surgery for UTUC prior to presentation to a tertiary care center which specializes in conservative endoscopic management for UTUC. Nevertheless, the potential for bilateral disease development in this special group must be considered when making treatment decisions and deserves future study. In general, UTUC cases in LS patients tend to present at younger ages, more often involve a primary tumor in the ureter versus the intrarenal collecting system and may have a tendency towards bilateral upper tract involvement more often when compared to sporadic UTUC cases (Table 9.3).

9.6 Screening for UTUC in Patients with Lynch Syndrome

The only malignancy in LS for which screening has been prospectively proven to decrease cancer specific mortality thus far, is in cases of CRC [40]. Currently, the official stance of HNPCC expert groups (sorely lacking urological representation) is that due to lack of evidence demonstrating benefit, there is no recommended surveillance protocol, outside of a research study, for UTUC in LS carrier patients at this time [15]. The National Comprehensive Cancer Network (NCCN) has posted surveillance guidelines in 2014, which state that practitioners may consider a yearly urinalysis in known LS carriers starting at age 25–30 years [2]. Others have instituted the use of voided urine cytology but this strategy alone has been retrospectively reported to have poor sensitivity and specificity for urothelial carcinoma in LS [41, 42]. Thus, no firm UTUC screening guidelines based on high quality evidence exist at this time.

The absence of level-one evidence on how to effectively screen for other LS malignancies, aside from CRC, is due to small numbers of identified patients. This is likely secondary to lack of awareness and the inability to recognize LS cases not only among the medical community as a whole, but especially within subspecialty groups that may see LS-related malignancies. There is literature suggesting that we are missing a significant number of UTUC patients with LS trait. Given the relative limited sensitivity of Amsterdam Criteria II for diagnosis of LS being 72 % [43], the members of the French collaborative national database on UTUC applied less stringent, but still well thought out, criteria to a cohort of 1,122 patients with UTUC in their database comprising a 15 year experience among 17 French institutions. The group reported that 239 patients (21 % of the database) with UTUC originally classified as sporadic may actually be hereditary in nature [44]. They presented a patient-screening tool to be used by all urologists in order to better identify any new patient with UTUC as a potential candidate for having an underlying hereditary etiology. This tool simply relies heavily on personal and familial history of LS malignancies but also very thoughtfully screens for any newly diagnosed UTUC patient less than 60 years of age. The French authors initially suggested this same type of screening-tool in 2004 after a retrospective study on NU specimens applying microsatellite instability (MSI) testing led to further investigation with mutational analysis and discovery of MSH-2 mutation in a proportion of consecutive UTUC patients not meeting Amsterdam Criteria II [45].

The retrospective but nevertheless repetitive trend in the literature for LS-associated UTUC cases to mostly involve mutations of the MSH-2 gene has led to the concept of risk stratification for screening LS carriers for UTUC [46]. According to the literature available, it would seem the LS patients most at risk for UTUC development are carriers of MSH-2 mutations and those with family history of UTUC. For now, any potential screening protocol for UTUC in LS patients or their potentially affected family members will rest on expert opinion. The production of level-one evidence for screening this population for UTUC will require awareness among all urologists to identify these patients and send them for genetic counseling. International collaboration and an agreed upon screening protocol with follow-up will be necessary to identify an effective screening strategy. This is a lofty but worthwhile goal given the fact that LS patients with UTUC present at younger ages and may be more susceptible to bilateral UTUC development.

References

1. Margulis V, Shariat SF, Matin SF, Kamat AM, Zigeuner R, Kikuchi E, Lotan Y, Weizer A, Raman JD, Wood CG. Outcomes of radical nephroureterectomy: a series from the upper tract urothelial carcinoma collaboration. Cancer. 2009;115:1224–33.

2. National Comprehensive Cancer Network Clinical Practice Guidelines in Oncology (NCCN guidelines): Lynch Syndrome V.2.2014.

3. Shariat SF, Favaretto RL, Gupta A, et al. Gender differences in radical nephroureterectomy for upper tract urothelial carcinoma. World J Urol. 2011;29:481–6.

4. Holmang S, Johansson SL. Bilateral metachronous ureteral and renal pelvic carcinomas: incidence, clinical presentation, histopathology, treatment and outcome. J Urol. 2006;175:69–73.

5. Hall MC, Womak S, Sagalosky AI, Carmody T, Erickstad MD, Roehrborn CG. Prognostic factors, recurrence, and survival in transitional cell carcinoma of the upper urinary tract: 30 year experience in 252 patients. Urology. 1998;52:594–601.

6. Grasso M, Fishman AI, Cohen J, et al. Ureteroscopic and extirpative treatment of upper urinary tract urothelial carcinoma: a 15-year comprehensive review of 160 consecutive patients. BJU Int. 2012;110: 1618–26.

7. Fang D, Xiong G, Li X, et al. Incidence, characteristics, treatment strategies and oncological outcomes of synchronous bilateral upper tract urothelial carcinoma in the Chinese population. Urol Oncol. 2014. pii: S1078-1439(14)00224-5. doi:10.1016/j.urolonc.2014.07.001. [Epub ahead of print].

8. Luo HL, Kang CH, Chen YT, Chuang YC, Lee WC, Cheng YT, Chiang PH. Diagnostic ureteroscopy independently correlates with intravesical recurrence after nephroureterectomy for upper urinary tract urothelial carcinoma. Ann Surg Oncol. 2013;20(9):3121–9.

9. Li CC, Chang TH, Wu WJ, et al. Significant predictive factors for prognosis of primary upper urinary tract cancer after radical nephroureterectomy in Taiwanese patients. Eur Urol. 2008;54:1127–35.

10. Milenkovic-Petronic D, Milojevic B, Djokic M, et al. The impact of tumor size on outcomes in patients with upper urinary tract urothelial carcinoma. Int Urol Nephrol. 2014;46:563–9.

11. Watson P, Vasen HF, Mecklin JP, et al. The risk of extra-colonic, extra-endometrial cancer in the Lynch syndrome. Int J Cancer. 2008;123:444–9.

12. Crockett DG, Wagner DG, Holmang S, et al. Upper urinary tract carcinoma in lynch syndrome cases. J Urol. 2011;185:1627–30.

13. Hubosky SG, Boman BM, Charles S, et al. Ureteroscopic management of upper tract urothelial carcinoma (UTUC) in patients with Lynch Syndrome (hereditary nonpolyposis colorectal cancer syndrome). BJU Int. 2013;112(6):813–9.

14. Hampel H, de la Chapelle A. How do we approach the goal of identifying everybody with Lynch Syndrome? Fam Cancer. 2013;12:313–7.

15. Vasen HF, Blacno I, Aktan-Collan K, et al. Revised guidelines for the clinical management of Lynch syndrome (HNPCC): recommendations by a group of European experts. Gut. 2013;62:812–23.

16. Vasen HF, Wijnen J, Menko FH, et al. Cancer risk in families with hereditary nonpolyposis colorectal cancer diagnosed by mutation analysis. Gastroenterology. 1996;110:1020–7.

17. Huben RP, Mounzer AM, Murphy GP. Tumor grade and stage as prognostic variables in upper tract urothelial tumors. Cancer. 1988;62:2016–20.

18. McLaughlin JK, Silverman DT, Hsing AW, et al. Cigarette smoking and cancers of the renal pelvis and ureter. Cancer Res. 1992;52:254–7.

19. Jensen OM, Knudsen JB, McLaughlin JK, Sorensen BL. The Copenhagen case-control study of renal pelvis and ureter cancer: role of smoking and occupational exposures. Int J Cancer. 1988;41:557–61.

20. Nortier JL, Muniz Martinez MZ, Schmeiser HH, et al. Urothelial carcinoma associated with the use of a Chinese herb (Aristolochia fangchi). N Engl J Med. 2000;342:1686–92.

21. Hranjec T, Kovac A, Kos J, Mao W, Chen JJ, Grollman AP, et al. Endemic nephropathy: the case for chronic poisoning by aristolochia. Croat Med J. 2005;46: 116–25.

22. Matin SF, Shariat SF, Milowsky MI, Hansel DE, Kassouf W, Koppie T, Bajorin D, Grollman AP. Highlights from the first symposium on upper tract urothelial carcinoma. Urol Oncol. 2014;32(3): 309–16.

23. Warthin AS. Hereditary with reference to carcinoma as shown by the study of the cases examined in the pathological laboratory of the University of Michigan, 1895–1913. Arch Intern Med. 1913;12:546–55.

24. Lynch HT, Krush AJ. Cancer family "G" revisited: 1895–1970. Cancer. 1971;27:1505–11.

25. Vasen HF, Mecklin JP, Khan PM, et al. The International Collaborative Group on hereditary non-polyposis colorectal cancer (ICG-HNPCC). Dis Colon Rectum. 1991;34:424.

26. Fishel R, Lescoe MK, Rao MRS, Copeland NG, Jenkins NA, Garber J, Kane M, Kolodner R. The Human mutator gene homolog MSH2 and its association with hereditary nonpolyposis colon cancer. Cell. 1993;75:1027–38.

27. Nickolas P, Nicolaides NC, Wei Y-F, et al. Mutation of a mutL homolog in hereditary colon cancer. Science. 1994;263(5153):1625–9.

28. Watson P, Lynch HT. Extracolonic cancer in hereditary nonpolyposis colorectal cancer. Cancer. 1993;71: 677–85.

29. Vasen HF, Watson P, Mecklin JP, et al. New clinical criteria for hereditary nonpolyposis colorectal cancer (HNPCC, Lynch syndrome) proposed by the International Collaborative group on HNPCC. Gastroenterology. 1999;116:1453–6.

30. Rodriguez-Bigas MA, Boland CR, Hamilton SR, et al. A National Cancer Institute Workshop on hereditary nonpolyposis colorectal cancer syndrome: meeting highlights and Bethesda Guidelines. J Natl Cancer Inst. 1997;89(23):1758–62.

31. Lindor NM, Petersen GM, Hadley DW, et al. Recommendations for the care of individuals with an inherited predisposition to Lynch syndrome. JAMA. 2006;296(12):1507–17.

32. Lynch HT, de la Chapelle A. Hereditary colorectal cancer. N Engl J Med. 2003;348:919–32.

33. Jass JR, Stewart SM. Evolution of hereditary non-polyposis colorectal cancer. Gut. 1992;33:783–6.

34. Watson P, Lin K, Rodriguez-Bigas MA, et al. Colorectal carcinoma survival among hereditary nonpolyposis colorectal cancer family members. Cancer. 1998;83:259–66.

35. Sankila R, Aaltonen LA, Jarvinen HJ, et al. Better survival rates in patients with MLH1-associated hereditary colorectal cancer. Gastroenterology. 1996;110:682–7.

36. Vasen HF, Mecklin JP, Khan PM, Lynch HT. The international collaborative group on HNPCC. Anticancer Res. 1994;14:1661–4.

37. Umar A, Boland CR, Terdiman JP, et al. Revised Bethesda Guidelines for hereditary nonpolyposis colorectal cancer (Lynch syndrome) and microsatellite instability. J Natl Cancer Inst. 2004;96:261–8.

38. Charbit L, Gendreau MC, Mee S, et al. Tumors of the upper urinary tract: 10 years experience. J Urol. 1991;146:1243–6.

39. Sijmons RH, Kiemeney LA, Witjes JA, et al. Urinary tract cancer and hereditary nonpolyposis colorectal cancer: risks and screening options. J Urol. 1998; 160:466–70.

40. Jarvinen HJ, Aarnio M, Mustonen H, et al. Controlled 15-year trial on screening for colorectal cancer in families with hereditary nonpolyposis colorectal cancer. Gastroenterology. 2000;118:829–34.

41. Myrhoj T, Andersen MB, Bernstein I. Screening for urinary tract cancer with urine cytology in Lynch syndrome and familial colorectal cancer. Fam Cancer. 2008;7:303–7.

42. Bernstein IT, Myrhoj T. Surveillance for urinary tract cancer in Lynch syndrome. Fam Cancer. 2013;12: 279–84.

43. Lynch HT, Boland CR, Rodriguez-Bigas MA, et al. Who should be sent for genetic testing in hereditary colorectal cancer syndromes? J Clin Oncol. 2007;25: 3534–42.

44. Audenet F, Colin P, Yates DR, et al. A proportion of hereditary upper tract urothelial carcinomas are misclassified as sporadic according to a multi-institutional database analysis: proposal of patient-specific risk identification tool. BJU Int. 2012;110:E583–9.

45. Rouprot M, Catto J, Coulet F, et al. Microsatellite instability as indicator of MSH2 gene mutation in patients with upper urinary tract transitional cell carcinoma. J Med Genet. 2004;41, e91.

46. Archer P, Kiela G, Thomas K, et al. Towards a rational strategy for the surveillance of patients with Lynch syndrome (hereditary non-polyposis colon cancer) for upper tract transitional cell carcinoma. BJU Int. 2010;106:300–2.

Christopher B. Anderson[$], John E. Musser[$],
John P. Sfakianos, and Harry W. Herr

10.1 Introduction

Following treatment for urothelial carcinoma of the bladder (UCB), patients are at risk for urothelial recurrence in the bladder, urethra and upper tracts. This may be due to a field effect in the urothelium or implantation of malignant cells shed from the primary tumor [1]. Conversely, following treatment for upper tract urothelial carcinomas (UTUC) there is a 13–54 % and 6 % risk of recurrence in the bladder and contralateral upper tract, respectively [2]. Theoretical causes for intravesical recurrence following treatment for UTUC include tumor cell shedding during surgery, angiogenic factors released into the bladder as a consequence of the bladder incision, and a compromised immune status due to surgery [3]. Because there is a risk of UTUC after treatment for UCB, and UCB after treatment for UTUC, long-term surveillance of the urothelium is necessary in patients with a history of urothelial carcinoma.

[$] Author contributed equally with all other contributors.

C.B. Anderson, MD • H.W. Herr, MD (✉)
Urology Service, Department of Surgery, Memorial
Sloan Kettering Cancer Center, 1275 York Avenue,
New York, NY 10065, USA
e-mail: cbanderson2014@gmail.com; herrh@mskcc.org

J.E. Musser, MD • J.P. Sfakianos, MD
Department of Surgery, Memorial Sloan Kettering
Cancer Center, 1275 York Avenue,
New York, NY 10065, USA
e-mail: musser89@gmail.com; johnsfak@gmail.com

10.2 Upper Tract Recurrence After Treatment for Urothelial Carcinoma of the Bladder

10.2.1 Upper Tract Recurrences After the Treatment of Non-muscle Invasive Bladder Cancer

Approximately 80 % of patients diagnosed with UCB have non-muscle invasive disease [1]. While non-muscle invasive bladder cancer (NIMBC) is associated with a relatively low risk of cancer-specific mortality, it has a high likelihood of local recurrence [4].

Upper tract imaging is required at the time of bladder cancer diagnosis to rule out synchronous upper tract tumors, which are seen in 1–4 % of patients [5–10]. Among 28 bladder cancer patients diagnosed with synchronous upper tract tumors, nearly half of the upper tract tumors were muscle invasive, half were located in the ureter, and there was a high correlation between bladder tumor grade and upper tract tumor grade [9]. Patients with tumors located in the trigone may be at particularly high risk for synchronous upper tract tumors.

The risk of metachronous upper tract recurrence (UTR) in patients with NIMBC ranges from 0.6 to 25 %, depending on disease characteristics (Table 10.1) [10, 11, 12–16]. Upper tract recurrences are generally diagnosed 3–5 years

© Springer International Publishing Switzerland 2015
M. Grasso III, D.H. Bagley (eds.), *Upper Urinary Tract Urothelial Carcinoma*,
DOI 10.1007/978-3-319-13869-5_10

Table 10.1 Upper tract recurrences after treatment for NIMBC

Study	Number of patients	Median follow-up (months)	Cohort	UTR prevalence	Median time to UTR (months)	UTR risk factors	UTR location	UTR characteristics
Solsanaa et al. [10]	138	86	NIMBC with CIS	24.6 % CIS: 21.2 % No CIS: 2.3 %	38 CIS: 38 (0–56) [mean] No CIS: 44 (3–122) [mean]	Involvement of prostatic urethra	12 % renal pelvis 88 % distal ureter 32 % bilateral	68 % non-invasive 20 % invasive 12 % unknown
Herr [12]	307	146 (120–216)	NIMBC treated with BCG	25 %	56 (12–181)	Retained bladder	44 % renal pelvis 56 % ureter	23 % non-invasive 77 % invasive
Hurle et al. [13]	591	80–92 (27–143)	All NIMBC	4 % Low risk: 0.9 % Intermediate risk: 2.2 % High risk: 9.8 %	80 (16–230) Low risk: 80, 91 Intermediate risk: 52 (16–109) High risk: 49 (16–107)	Grade Stage CIS Multifocality Recurrent IVC failure	48 % renal pelvis 36 % distal ureter 16 % multifocal	60 % non-invasive 40 % invasive
Millan-Rodriguez et al. [14]	1,529		All NIMBC	2.6 % Low risk: 0.6 % Intermediate risk: 1.8 % High risk: 4.1 %	Low risk: 122 Intermediate risk: 47 (27–67) High risk: 39 (10–68)	Grade Stage CIS Multifocality	41 % renal pelvis 41 % ureter 18 % multifocal	47 % non-invasive 33 % invasive 20 % unknown
Canales et al. [15]	375	58 (14–176)	Ta only	3.4 % Low risk:1.8 % High risk: 8.9 %	22 months [mean] Low risk: 43 [mean] High risk: 24 [mean]	≥2 prior intravesical recurrences <12 months between intravesical recurrences	77 % renal pelvis 23 % ureter	77 % non-invasive 23 % invasive
Wright et al. [20]	99,388		All bladder cancer (85 % NIMBC)	0.8 %	33	Grade CIS Location Cystectomy	45 % renal pelvis 54 % ureter	55–59 % localized 40–51 % poorly differentiated
Sternberg et al. [16]	935	66	All NIMBC	5.4 %	≤60 months: 57 % recurred >60 months: 43 % recurred	Stage CIS		

UTR upper tract recurrence, *NIMBC* non-muscle invasive bladder cancer, *CIS* carcinoma in situ, *BCG* Bacille Calmette-Guerin, *IVC* intravesical chemotherapy after NIMBC diagnosis and the entire upper tract is at risk for developing an UTR, with approximately half occuring in the renal pelvis, half in the ureter, and 20 % multifocal.

Risk Factors

Patients with T1 NIMBC had nearly double the risk of UTR at 10 years compared to patients with Ta, and patients with at least two prior NIMBC recurrences or an duration of less than 12 months between recurrences had a fivefold higher rate of UTR than those without either (8.9 % vs. 1.8 %) [15, 16]. Other potential risks include vesicoureteral reflux and occupational exposure, although their relative importance is less certain [17–19].

One study stratified patients into low, intermediate and high risk groups according to NIMBC grade, stage, multifocality and presence of CIS, and found UTRs in 0.6, 1.8 and 4.1 % of the patients in each respective risk group [14]. All UTRs occurred in patients who had at least one prior intravesical recurrence, and bladder tumor multifocality tripled the risk. A similar study estimated risk of UTR according to several clinical risk factors [13]. Patients with primary, solitary and low grade NIMBC had a 0.9 % prevalence of UTR, while those with recurrent or multifocal tumors had a 2.2 % prevalence. The highest risk group had a UTR prevalence of 9.8 % and included patients with CIS or high grade tumors and those who failed prior intravesical chemotherapy.

Patients with NIMBC and associated CIS, and those treated intravesical bacillus Calmette Guérin (BCG) are a particurlarly high risk group with up to a 25 % risk of UTR [10, 12]. At 5, 10 and 15 years, patients treated with BCG had a 13, 28 and 38 % cumulative risk of UTR and patients with CIS may have a ten-fold increased risk as compared to patients without CIS. Patients with bladder CIS are also more likely to develop bilateral UTRs, and those with disease in the prostatic urethra have particularly poor outcomes [10].

In an analysis of nearly 100,000 bladder cancer patients from the SEER registry, of whom 85 % had NIMBC, 0.8 % were diagnosed with an UTR [20]. Upper tract recurrences were more common in patients with NIMBC, and risk factors included the presence of bladder CIS, higher grade bladder tumors and bladder tumors located at the ureteral orifice, trigone or bladder neck.

Upper tract recurrences are relatively late events, thus length of follow-up is strongly influential on the risk of developing an UTR. The prevalence of UTR in high risk patients is less than 10 % after 4 years, but may be at least 25 % after 12 years [12–14]. Approximately half of the UTRs occur more than 5 years after NIMBC diagnosis, and some can occur as late as 15 years [12, 16]. Given the length to time needed to develop UTRs and because UTRs typically occur in patients who have not experienced a competing event, such as metastatsis or death, the longer patients are followed in absence of a competing event, the more likely they are to experience an UTR. This explains the seemingly paradoxical observation that patients with invasive bladder tumors and those who have radical cystectomy (RC) have lower rates of UTR [12, 20]. These patients have a higher risk of competing events due to thier aggressive disease, and fewer are at-risk for developing an UTR.

Outcomes

While characteristics of UTRs vary across studies, patients with higher risk bladder tumors tend to develop more aggressive upper tract tumors (Table 10.1). Nearly 80 % of UTRs were muscle invasive in patients with high risk NIMBC, while only 23–32 % were invasive in patients with lower risk tumors [12–15]. From 60 to 96 % of patients with UTRs require aggressive treatment with nephroureterectomy or segmental ureterectomy, although endoscopic treatment can be an option for some [13–15]. Although some have suggested no difference in survival for patients with versus without UTRs [10], 20–32 % will ultimately die from metastastatic disease [12, 13, 15]. Those who die are generally patients with high risk NIMBC and high grade UTRs.

Surveillance After NIMBC Treatment

There is conflicting evidence about whether UTRs are more often diagnosed on surveillance studies or due to the onset of symptoms, however there is no evidence that detecting an asymptomatic UTR translates to better patient outcomes [13, 15, 16]. One series found that approximately two-thirds of UTRs were detected symptomatically and only a quarter were diagnosed asymptomatically on surveillance imaging [16]. CT urography was used most commonly for upper tract surveillance, but proved unnecessary for most patients as the vast majority of UTRs could have been diagnosed with ultrasound or urine cytology. In fact, only 3 out of 51 (6 %) UTRs would have been missed if surveillance CT urography had not been routinely performed on asymptomatic patients.

All professional guidelines recommend a risk stratified approach to upper tract surveillance in asymptomatic patients with a history fo NIMBC (Table 10.2) [5–7, 21]. Because half of all recurrences are detected 5 years after NIMBC diagnosis and this risk does not decrease over time, long-term surveillance in high risk patients is necessary [10–12, 15, 16, 22]. The most common imaging modality is CT urography, which effectively images the renal parenchyma and upper

urinary tracts. Other modalities include intravenous pyelography, MR urography, renal ultrasound with retrograde pyelogram and ureteroscopy. Patients with symptoms or positive urinary cytology in the absence of cystoscopic findings should receive upper tract imaging.

10.2.2 Upper Tract Recurrences After Radical Cystectomy

Up to 50 % of patients experience recurrence of urothelial carcinoma following RC, most commonly within 2 years of surgery at metastatic sites within the abdomen and pelvis, chest and bone [23–25]. If patients do not recurr during this early period, there is still an 8 % risk of disease recurrence, most commonly in the upper urinary tracts [24]. Most contemporary series report the risk of UTR following RC between 2 and 6 % with a time to recurrence of 2–3 years (Table 10.3) [10, 25–34]. Over half of UTRs occur in the renal pelvis, up to a quarter are multifocal, and recurrences at the ureteroileal anastomosis are rare [27–31, 33].

Table 10.2 Professional guideline recommendations for upper tract surveillance in asymptomatic patients after NIMBC treatment

NCCN [6]		AUA [7, 88]		EAU [5]	
Risk group	Upper tract Imaging[a]	Risk group[b]	Upper tract Imaging	Risk group[c]	Upper tract Imaging[d]
Ta LG	None	Low risk	None	Low risk	None
Ta HG	Consider every 1–2 years	Intermediate risk	Consider	Intermediate risk	None
T1 LG	None	High risk	Annually for 2 years, then lengthen interval	High risk	Annually
T1 HG	Consider every 1–2 years				
Any Tis	Consider every 1–2 years				

NCCN National Comprehensive Cancer Network, *AUA* American Urological Association, *EAU* European Association of Urology, *LG* low grade, *CIS* carcinoma *in situ*

Intermediate risk: Any tumors not defined by low or high risk

High risk: Any of the following – T1, high grade, presence of CIS, multiple and recurrent and large (>3 cm) LGTa tumors

[a]Modalities include intravenous pyelogram, CT urography, renal ultrasound with retrograde pyelogram, ureteroscopy, or MR urogram

[b]Low risk: solitary LGTa

[c]Low risk: primary, solitary, small (<3 cm) LGTa tumors with no CIS

[d]CT urogram or intravenous pyelogram

Table 10.3 Upper tract recurrence following radical cystectomy

Study	Number of patients	Median follow-up (months)	UTR prevalence	Median time to UTR (months)	UTR risk factors
Kenworthy et al. [28]	430		2.6 %	40 (9–56)	Distal ureteral involvement
Solsana et al. [10]	225		CIS: 17.4 % No CIS: 3.9 %	CIS: 18 No CIS: 28	CIS
Sved et al. [30]	235	42 [mean]	2 %	40 (16–60) [mean]	Prostatic urethral involvement
Sanderson et al. [29]	1,069	124 (4–222)	2.5 %	40 (5–112)	Superficial urethral involvement
Tran et al. [32]	1,329	38 (17–70)	6 %	25 (1–107)	Distal ureteral involvement
Furukawa et al. [27]	583	42 (7–77)	2.1 %	30 (5–71)	
Meissner et al. [41]	322		4.7 %	31 (12–72)	
Volkmer et al. [33]	1,420		1.8 %	39 (4–142)	CIS Recurrent bladder tumor RC for NIMBC Distal ureteral involvement
Umbreit et al. [25]	1,388	172	4.8 %	37 (2–174)	Multifocality Positive ureteral margin pT4 Gross hematuria
Takayanagi et al. [31]	362	48 (0–214)	3 %	48 (12–79)	CIS Positive ureteral margin Urethral involvement
Perlis et al. [34]	574	45	4 %	28 (8–96)	

CIS carcinoma *in situ, NIBMC* non-muscle invasive bladder cancer

Risk Factors

Approximately 10 % of RC specimens demonstrate involvement of the distal ureter with carcinoma on final pathology, and this finding is associated with a two to sixfold increased risk of UTR [25, 28, 32, 33]. On one study, 16 % of RC patients with ureteral involvement were diagnosed with UTR a 5 years comapred to 5 % without ureteral involvement [32].

The male and female urethra can be involved with urothelial carcinoma in 15 % and 63 % of RC specimens, respectively [29]. Patients with superficial urethral involvement have a higher 10 year risk of UTR compared to those without it (15–19 % vs. 3–4 %), and some suggest that urethral involvement is a stronger predictor of UTR than ureteral involvement [29, 31]. As expected,

prostatic stromal invoement is not consistently associated with an increased risk of UTR, as these patients are more likely to experience cancer-speficic mortality and few are at risk to develop UTR [29].

Bladder tumor characteristics that reflect the presence of aggressive, recurrent or refractory disease increase the risk of UTR. Multifocality and a history of recurrent NIMBC were associated with a two to three times increased risk of UTR [25, 33], and RC patients with NIMBC have a higher risk of UTR than RC patients with invasive disease [33]. Bladder CIS is identified up to 50 % of RC specimens and is associated with a two to sixfold increased risk of UTR [10, 29, 31–33]. Interestingly, bladder CIS triples the risk of ureteral involvement [32].

A recent meta-analysis of over 13,000 patients reported a 0.8–6.4 % prevalence of UTR after RC [35]. On multivariable analysis, lower tumor grade, RC for NIMBC, bladder CIS, positive ureteral margin, positive urethral margin, a history of UTUC and pathologically negative lymph nodes were independendtly associated with an increased risk of UTR. These results mirror those from individual studies and suggest that bladder tumor characteristics associated with locally aggressive and recurrent disease, but not lethal disease, predict higher rates of UTR.

Similar to UTRs after NIMBC, one of the strongest risk factors for UTR after RC is length of follow-up. As UTR is a relatively late event, patients who develop metastatic disease in the first years following RC usually die and are not at risk to develop UTR. Therefore, RC patients with longer follow-up who do not have a competing event are at an increased risk of UTR. Importantly, this risk of does not decrease over time [22, 32].

Use of Ureteral Frozen Section

Because ureteral involvement is a strong risk factor for UTR, many surgeons routinely send an intraoperative frozen section examination (FSE) of the disetal ureter and perform a stepwise resection in effort to attain a negative margin. Proponents of this practice accept the need to perform a nephroureterectomy if necessary [36]. The utility of routine FSE was addressed in a large RC series where half of the patients had routine intraoperative ureteral FSE [37]. The sensitivty and specificity of FSE to detect ureteral involvement on final pathology was 75 % and 99 %, respectively, and a positive margin on final pathology nearly tripled the risk of UTR. However, most patients with postive FSE did not have enough ureteral length to warrant further step-sectioning, and those who did were infrequently converted to a negative margin on subsequent FSE. Ultimately, conversion from a positve FSE to a negative margin on final pathology did not eliminate the risk of UTR, and ureteral involvement was not associated with overall survival.

Other studies agree that FSE is accurate at detecting ureteral involvement and question its utility given the lack of evidence that ureteral involvement impacts survival, although it remains a topic of debate [36, 38–40]. A different RC series demonstrated that 82.6 % of 178 positive FSEs could be converted to a negative margin on final pathology with step-sectioning [39]. While ureteral involvement was not related to survival, and all patients with a positive FSE had an increased risk of UTR, those with a positive FSE who could be converted to a negative final margin had a slightly lower risk of UTR (HR 4.4, 95 % CI 2.6,7.4) than those who could not be converted to a negative final margin (HR 7.4, 95 % CI 4.3, 16.4).

Because of the pagetoid growth pattern of urothelial carcinoma, a negative FSE cannot rule out proximal upper tract involvement, and patients with a unilateral positive FSM can have a contralateral UTR [39]. With routine transection of the ureters at the common iliac artery, as few as 1.2 % of patients will have a positive ureteral margin on final pathology [38]. While FSE can identify ureteral involvement and may reduce the risk of UTR, it is an added expense that predicts a rare event and does not improve survival. At present, there is no strong evidence to support use of routine ureteral FSE. It is our practice to not send routine FSEs, but instead to perform high transection of the ureters with close monitoring of patients who have ureteral involvement on final pathology.

Outcomes

Upper tract recurrence following RC tends to be aggressive and have poor prognosis. Most patients with UTRs present with advanced stage and lymph node postive tumors, and as many as half present with metastatic disease [26, 27, 29, 31, 33]. Approximately 70 % of patients with UTRs after RC will die from urothelial carcinoma, and median survival is close to 1 year with less than 30 % alive at 5 years [26, 27, 29–31, 33]

Surveillance After RC

Surveillance regimens following RC include frequent office visits, cross-sectional imaging and urine cytology in the first 2–3 years and then at least annually thereafter. Still, some question the value of upper tract surveillance since 40–80 %

of UTRs present with a sign or symptom; most commonly gross hematuria, but also flank pain, renal failure, infection and weight loss [26, 28–31, 33]. Importantly, there is no obvious improvement in outcomes for patients who present with an asymptomatic versus symptomatic UTRs.

In one series of 15 UTRs after RC, half were diagnosed due to symptoms and there was no difference in survival between patients with an asymptomatic UTR found on surveillance and a symptomatic UTR [41]. Of the 1,064 surveillance intravenous pyelograms performed, only eight (0.75 %) were abnormal and led to the diagnosis of an asymptomatic UTR. Another study observed that while patients with asymptomatic distant recurrences tended to have improved survival compared to those with symptomatic distant recurrences, this was not seen for patients with urothelial recurrences, including UTRs [42]. Still, patients with UTRs detected asymptomatically on routine surveillance may have better survival compared to those who presented symptomatically (1.6 vs. 3.7 years), although this difference was not significant (p=0.6) [29].

Urinary biomarkers are also used to monitor for urothelial recurrence. Since the majority of UTRs are high grade, urinary cytology is theoretically a useful test. The sensitivity of urinary cytology for detecting UTRs ranges from 40 % to 100 %, but as many as 90 % of positive cytologies are falsely positive [41, 43]. In a cohort 278 RC patients, only one out of nearly 500 surveillance urine cyologies helped diagnose a UTR that would not have been otherwise detected due to symptoms or abnormal imaging [43]. Fluoroesence *in situ* hybridization has a 86 % sensitivity and 87 % specificity for detecting UTRs after RC, with a similarly low positive predictive value as cytology [43].

Both urinary cytology and upper tract imaging have low yields for detecting UTR when performed on asymptomatic patients, with 2,000 and 800 patients needed to be screened with cytology and upper tract imaging, respectively, to detect one UTR [35]. While routine cross-sectional imaging may be useful to detect distant recurrences and other postoperative complications, it is currently unknown whether diagnosing an asymptomatic UTR has a more favorable prognosis than one detected symptomatically [44].

A risk-stratified surveillance strategy may improve yield and reduce unnecessary tests. Considering the presence of CIS, recurrent bladder cancer, RC for NIMBC and distal ureteral involvement, patients who had 0, 1–2 and 3–4 of these findings had a 15 year UTR risk of 0.8 %, 8.2 % and 13.1 %, respectively [33]. If all RC patients were imaged annually for 5 years, the chance of diagnosing a UTR in patients with 0, 1–2 and 3–4 risk factors was 1:432, 1:93 and 1:53, respectively. Similarly, when stratifying patients based on the presence of either urethral involvement or bladder CIS, the 5-year prevalence of UTR for patients with either risk present versus neither was 12 % versus 0.9 % [31].

The NCCN currently offers the only guideline recommendations for surveillance following RC. They recommend cross-sectional and upper tract imaging every 3–6 months for 5 years, then as clinically indicated depending on the risk of recurrence [6]. Since UTRs may occur many years after RC and, in the absence of a competing event, the risk does not decrease over time, high risk patients require lifelong surveillance [22, 32]. Going forward, studies are needed to examine whether UTR surveillance strategies that are less reliant on frequent cross-sectional imaging, but instead use urinary cytology, renal ultrasound and physical examination, have comparable safety and effectiveness, both for patients with native bladders as well as after RC.

10.3 Bladder Recurrence Following Treatment for Upper Tract Urothelial Carcinoma

Risk Factors

Identification of risk factors for intravesical recurrence following treatment of UTUC can help guide post-treatment surveillance regimens, and identify patients who would benefit most from adjuvant intravesical treatments. While treatment of intravesical recurrences is usually

Table 10.4 Prevalence and risk factors for bladder recurrence after treatment of UTUC

Study	Number of patients	Median follow-up (months)	Intravesical recurrence rate (%)	Risks for intravesical recurrence
Sakamoto et al. (1991) [89]	53		36	Synchronous bladder tumor Multiple UTUC tumors
Krough et al. (1991) [59]	198		36	UTUC location
Mukamel et al. (1994) [50]	69		48	UTUC grade UTUC multifocality
Hall et al. (1998) [90]	252	64	13	UTUC stage UTUC treatment modality
Hisataki et al. (2000) [48]	69	53	35	UTUC stage
Koga et al. (2001) [51]	85	35	34	Female gender Adjuvant systemic chemotherapy Incomplete ureterectomy
Kang et al. (2003) [2]	189	91	31	UTUC mutifocality
Matsui et al. (2005) [46]	89	40	42	UTUC mutifocality UTUC stage UTUC tumor size Surgical approach
Raman et al. (2005) [53]	103	39	50	Previous bladder cancer
Zigeuner et al. (2006) [49]	191	33	27	UTUC location UTUC grade
Novara et al. (2008) [54]	231	38	47	Previous bladder cancer
Li et al. (2008) [52]	260	56	34	Male gender Renal insufficiency
Pieras et al. (2010) [45]	79	71	54	UTUC tumor size UTUC with CIS
Xylinas et al. (2014) [47]	2681	58	22	Endoscopic approach to distal ureter UTUC with CIS

UTUC upper urinary tract carcinoma, *CIS* carcinoma *in situ*

successful, the required therapy is highly dependent on stage at diagnosis, making early detection critical.

Numerous studies have examined risk factors for intravesical recurrence after nephroureterectomy (NU) for UTUC (Table 10.4). Upper tract tumor risk factors include size [45, 46], presence of upper tract CIS [45, 47], stage [46, 48], grade [49, 50], location [49], and multifocality [2, 46]. Other risk factors are gender [51, 52], incomplete bladder cuff excision [51], a prior history of bladder tumors [53, 54], and surgical approach [46, 47].

Most reports agree that UTUC multifocality and prior history of bladder cancer confer a higher risk of intravesical recurrence after treatment of UTUC. In a large multi-institutional series, upper tract tumor multifocality and a history of bladder cancer each nearly doubled the risk of intravesical recurrence after NU on multivariable analysis [55]. Additionally, there was a significantly higher risk of intravesical recurrence in patients treated with laparoscopic NU as compared to an open approach. However, other reports have indicated similar oncologic efficacy between laparoscopic and open approaches [56–58].

Other studies have reported that UTUCs located in the ureter had a higher risk of intravesical recurrence than those located more proximally [49, 59]. Any manipulation of the ureter and collecting system during NU prior to ligation of the distal ureter can shed tumor cells into the bladder, and UTUCs located more distally may have a greater tendency to shed cells.

The risk for intravesical recurrence after treatment of UTUC is highest several years after treatment, and studies with longer follow-up tend to report higher intravesical recurrence rates. While Xylinas et al. identified a 35 % prevalence of intravesical recurrence, many of their patients had limited follow-up [55]. Actuarial intravesical recurrence-free survival at 5 years was 45 % reinforcing the need for long-term surveillance.

Prevention

I. Management of Distal Ureter

Given the high incidence of intravesical recurrence after NU, there is an interest in preventative strategies. Resection of the entire ureter including intramural portion and bladder cuff at the time of NU for UTUC was first described by Kimball and Ferris in 1934, and is still considered necessary to optimize oncologic efficacy [60]. A transvesical approach is considered the gold standard, but several new techniques have been described.

The purported advantage of endoscopic and laparoscopic approaches to the distal ureter is

to minimize morbidity, especially when combined with a minimally invasive approach to NU. However, no study has demonstrated a clear advantage any one technique. Still, it is well accepted that failure to remove the entire ureter puts the patient at an unacceptable risk for distal ureteral recurrence, and there is some evidence that these techniques impact the risk of intravesical recurrence. In a comparison of transvesical, extravesical and endoscopic approaches to the distal ureter at the time of NU, the endoscopic approach was associated with higher intravesical recurrence rates (Fig. 10.1) [47].

It may be possible reduce intravesical recurrence rates following NU by early ligation or detachment of the distal ureter. This theoretically prevents shedding of tumor cells into the bladder during manipulation of the kidney and ureter. In one retrospective series, intravesical recurrence rates were compared between patients who underwent endoscopic detachment of the ureter prior to NU and patients whose kidney and ureters were completely mobilized first [61]. While the difference was not statistically significant, patients who underwent early endoscopic detachment of the ureter had a slightly lower risk of bladder recurrence (34.5 % vs. 39 %). On theoretical disadvantage to

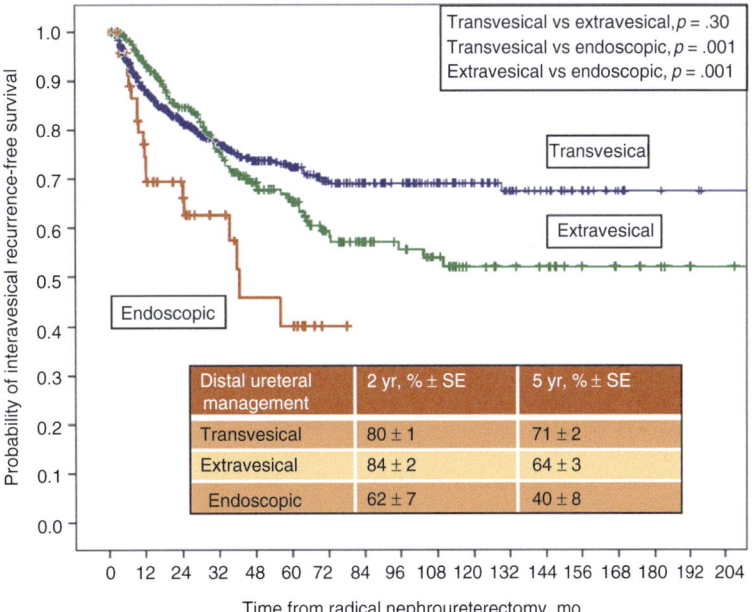

Fig. 10.1 Intravesical recurrence according to technique used to manage the distal ureter at the time of nephroureterectomy (Ref. [47], Reprinted with permission from Elsevier)

early endoscopic detachment is retroperitoneal tumor dissemination, and others have observed it to be associated with a higher risk of intravesical recurrence [47]. A randomized trial of 85 patients undergoing open NU found that early clipping of the distal ureter was associated with a decreased risk of intravesical recurrence [62]. Although the study was small, the relative ease with which one may place a clip on the distal ureter makes this an attractive technique.

II. Prophylactic Intravesical Chemotherapy

Given the success of a single instillation of intravesical chemotherapy to prevent recurrences after endoscopic resection for NIMBC [63–65], prophylactic intravesical chemotherapy was proposed as a measure to prevent intravesical recurrence after NU. Perioperative instillation is thought to treat microscopic tumor cells or prevent the implantation of tumors cells shed from the upper tract during surgery [3].

Three randomized trials have evaluated the efficacy of prophylactic intravesical chemotherapy following NU. The first randomized 25 patients to intravesical mitomycin C (MMC) plus cytosine arabinoside and no instillation [66]. Intravesical chemotherapy was initiated 1–2 weeks postoperatively and continued every 2 weeks for a total of 10 weeks and then monthly for 21 months. In all, patients received a total of 28 instillations over 2 years. Patients in the instillation group had lower intravesical recurrence rates at 1 (8 % vs.43 %) and 2 years (19 % vs. 43 %) translating into an eightfold lower risk (p=0.057). This risk appeared to be particularly lower in the first 100 days following NU. Still, this difference was not statistically significant, possibly due to the small sample size.

A multicenter study from the United Kingdom randomized 248 patients to 40 mg of intravesical MMC at the time of catheter removal (approximately 7–10 days following NU) or catheter removal without instillation [3]. On intention-to-treat analysis, a single postoperative dose of MMC reduced the incidence of intravesical recurrences during the first year after NU (17 %

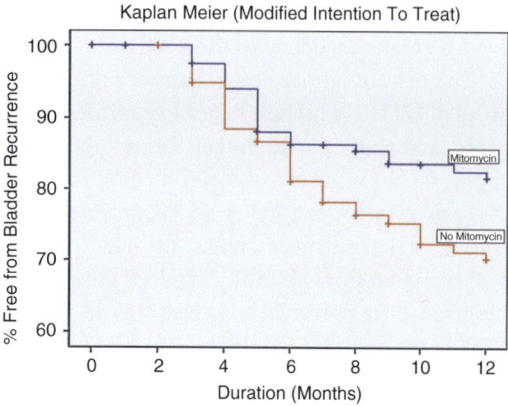

Fig. 10.2 Intravesical recurrence-free survival with versus without prophylactic intravesical mitomycin C following nephroureterectomy (Ref. [3], Reprinted with permission from Elsevier)

vs. 27 %, p=0.055), representing a 40 % relative risk reduction (Fig. 10.2). By per-protocol analysis, the recurrence rates were similar, but the difference was significant (p=0.03). Nine patients needed to be given intravesical MMC to prevent one intravesical recurrence.

The final study randomized 77 patients to a single 30 mg intravesical dose of pirarubicin (THP) within 48 h of NU or no intravesical treatment [67]. Patients that received THP had a significantly lower incidence of intravesical recurrence at one (16.9 % vs. 31.8 %) and two (16.9 % vs. 42.2 %) years as compared to the group that did not receive intravesical therapy (log-rank p=0.025, Fig. 10.3). The authors postulate that one of the benefits of THP over MMC is the shorter dwell time (30 min) compared to MMC (1 h).

These trials demonstrate promising results, but the precise timing, agent and dose of therapy to prevent bladder recurrences after NU remain unclear. Additionally, due to the small size of these studies, subgroup analyses were not possible and patient characteristics that predict a favorable response to treatment remain to be determined. While intravesical chemotherapy was generally well tolerated, there is a concern for extravasation and a risk of overtreatment. The adoption of prophylactic intravesical chemotherapy after NU has been relatively slow.

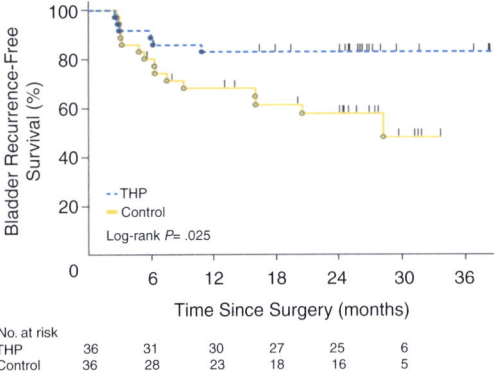

Surveillance and Prognosis

Intravesical recurrences after treatment for UTUC are common and have a better prognosis than distant recurrences. Most intravesical recurrences can be managed endoscopically, as more than 90 % of bladder recurrences were superficial and greater than 60 % were low to moderate grade [53]. Whether intravesical recurrences negatively impact survival in patients treated for UTUC is debatable. Mullerad et al. reported lower disease-specific survival after NU among those with metachronous intravesical recurrences, but others have suggested that intravesical recurrence after NU has no impact on survival [55, 68].

Stringent follow-up of patients after surgical treatment for UTUC is necessary to detect metachronous bladder tumors, and is supported by North American and European guidelines. The National Comprehensive Cancer Network advises cystoscopy every 3 months for the first year after treatment of UTUC, then at increasing intervals [6]. Similarly, cystoscopy and urinary cytology are advised at 3 months and then yearly for at least 5 years by the European Association of Urology [60]. Follow-up and surveillance after management of UTUC is discussed in Chap. 7.

10.4 Molecular Markers of Upper Tract Urothelial Carcinoma

Upper tract urothelial carcinoma and UCB have a similar histological appearance, although epidemiologic and clinicopathologic studies suggest that these tumors may be two distinct cancers. For instance, several risk factors are uniquely associated with UTUC, such as analgesic abuse and ingestion of aristolochic acid, an ingredient in some Chinese herbal remedies [69–71]. The most compelling evidence supporting the uniqueness of UTUC and UCB can be found at the molecular, genetic and epigenetic levels. Some of these differences hold prognostic significance.

There is a strong association between UTUC and Hereditary Non-Polyposis Colorectal Cancer (HNPCC), an autosomal dominant inherited genetic disease [72]. The genetic alterations associated with HNPCC are due to the presence of microsatellite instability (MSI) caused by deregulation of the DNA mismatch repair (MMR) system. Microsatellite instability stems from an inactivating germ-line mutation in the *hMSH2* (60 %), *hMLH1* (30 %) or *hMSH6* (5–8 %) genes, or from epigenetic changes leading to loss of function. Among 1,317 patients with HNPCC there was a 22-fold increased incidence of UTUC and a 10–15 year earlier onset compared to the general population [73]. However, a recent study observed that patients with HNPCC were also at higher risk of developing UCB [74]. More studies are needed to better understand the strength of association between inherited MSI and UTUC.

UTUCs may differ from UCB with regards to epigenetic changes. Among 280 primary sporadic urothelial carcinomas, promoter methylation for multiple key genes was more frequent in UTUC than in UCB (94 % vs. 76 %, p<0.0001), including hypermethylation of the *hMLH1* promoter (12 % vs. 1 %, p<0.001) [75]. UTUCs were more likely to have promoter methylation even when controlled for stage and grade. In addition, methylation at the *RASSF1A* and *DAPK* loci in both UTUC and UCB tumors was associated with disease progression (p <0.04).

Elevated microsatellite alteration at select tetranucleotides (EMAST) is another form of MSI that occurs in approximately 40 % of bladder tumors [76, 77]. One study found that UTUC tumors were less likely to have EMAST instability than UCB tumors (45 % vs 23 %, p = 0.009) [78]. However, UTUCs were more likely to have high-level MSI (MSI-H) mutations than UCB (13 % vs. 1 %, p = 0.003), but there was no difference in low-level MSI (MSI-L) mutations (14 % vs. 7 %, p = 0.2).

While UTUC and UCB differ in the expression of certain genes, both UCB and UTUC can have similar chromosomal aberrations. Loss of chromosome 9 is seen in 50 % of urothelial tumors. In particular, five regions in chromosome 9 may be involved in the development of both bladder and upper tract urothelial carcinoma (9p22p23, 9p11p13, 9p12~13, 9p21~22 and 9p34), each of which harbor tumor suppressor genes [79, 80]. In addition, gains in 1p36, 6p22, 7p, 8q2, 11q13, 17, 19q13 and 20q and losses in 4q, 5p, 6q, 9p, 13q have been associated with both UTUC and UCB [81–83]. Analysis of a small number of UTUCs showed losses at 2q, 8p, 9q, 11p, 13q, 17p and 18q and gains at 1q, 6p, 8q and 17q, which are similar to aberrations identified in UCB [79].

Some chromosomal abnormalities unique to UTUC may hold prognostic importance. In a series of 96 UTUCs after NU, gain in 20q13.2 was found in 63 % of patients using FISH analysis. In this series, the strongest predictor of intravesical recurrence following NU was a gain of 20q13.2. Furthermore, a gain in 20q13.2 predicted early (less than 18 months) intravesical recurrences, but was unrelated to late (more than 18 months) intravesical recurrence [84]. If confirmed, these findings may allow for improved risk stratification and aid in the selection of patients for adjuvant intravesical therapy or the development of risk-stratified surveillance schedules.

Genomic sequencing and expression profiling studies of UTUC tumors aim to identify biomarkers that may allow for risk stratified treatment and surveillance strategies, and hold promise for use with targeted therapies. In a series of 147 sporadic UTUCs and 105 UCBs, van Oers et al. used polymerase chain reaction to sequence three exons that coded for *FGFR3* [85]. They identified a similar rate of *FGFR3* mutations in UTUC and UCB tumors (48 % vs. 46 %), but found more mutations in ureteral compared to renal pelvis tumors (59 % vs. 39 %, p = 0.02). There was a significant improvement in disease-specific survival for patients with ureteral tumors who had mutations in *FGFR3*. Izquierdo et al. used real-time reverse transcriptase polymerase chain reaction to compare expression patters of 13 cancer related genes between UTUC tumors and controls [86]. Six genes (*BIRC5*, *FGFR3*, *KRT20*, *UPK2*, *FXYD3* and *hTERT*) were significantly overexpressed in UTUC, three genes (*AGR2*, *TP52* and *VEGF*) were significantly under expressed in UTUC, and the remaining four genes (*IGF2*, *EBF1*, *CDH1* and *HER2*) did not show any expression differences between groups. Zhang et al. used Affymetric GeneChip technology to perform expression profiling of upper tract and bladder tumors [87]. They found a small number of differentially expressed genes, including *CLCA2* (12-fold lower in bladder tumors) and *GABRE* (tenfold lower in bladder tumors) which are associated with diffusion of chloride ion binding and transport. They also identified 778 genes differentially expressed between normal renal pelvis urothelium from normal bladder urothelium, more than half of which were overexpressed in the normal renal pelvis urothelium and 15 were related to sodium transportation.

Conclusion

Urothelial recurrences are problematic events after treatment for bladder tumors and upper tract tumors. Bladder tumor risk factors for UTR include CIS, high stage and grade, receipt of prior BCG, and long follow-up without a competing event. Upper tract recurrences tend to occur several years after the treatment of the primary bladder tumor and patients at highest risk require lifelong upper tract surveillance. Following treatment of UTUC, patients with multifocal, high grade and high stage upper tract tumors are at highest risk for intravesical recurrence. Several preventative strategies exist, including intravesical chemotherapy and early ligation of the distal ureter. Intravesical surveillance should continue for several years after treatment for UTUC. There are several genetic biomarkers that are differentially expressed in UTUC, which may assist in surveillance risk stratification and hold promise for use with targeted therapies.

References

1. Wood DP (2012) Campbell-Walsh urology, editor-in-chief, AJ. Wein; [editors, Louis R. Kavoussi … et al.]. In: Wein AJ, Kavoussi LR, Campbell MF (eds). 10th edn. Philadelphia: Elsevier Saunders.
2. Kang CH, Yu TJ, Hsieh HH, Yang JW, Shu K, Huang CC, Chiang PH, Shiue YL. The development of bladder tumors and contralateral upper urinary tract tumors after primary transitional cell carcinoma of the upper urinary tract. Cancer. 2003;98(8):1620–6. doi:10.1002/cncr.11691.
3. O'Brien T, Ray E, Singh R, Coker B, Beard R, British Association of Urological Surgeons Section of Organization. Prevention of bladder tumours after nephroureterectomy for primary upper urinary tract urothelial carcinoma: a prospective, multicentre, randomised clinical trial of a single postoperative intravesical dose of mitomycin C (the ODMIT-C Trial). Eur Urol. 2011;60(4):703–10. doi:10.1016/j.eururo.2011.05.064.
4. Siegel R, Ma J, Zou Z, Jemal A. Cancer statistics, 2014. CA A Cancer J Clin. 2014;64(1):9–29. doi:10.3322/caac.21208.
5. Babjuk M, Burger M, Zigeuner R, Shariat SF, van Rhijn BW, Comperat E, Sylvester RJ, Kaasinen E, Bohle A, Palou Redorta J, Roupret M. EAU guidelines on non-muscle-invasive urothelial carcinoma of the bladder: update 2013. Eur Urol. 2013;64(4):639–53. doi:10.1016/j.eururo.2013.06.003.
6. Clark PE, Agarwal N, Biagioli MC, Eisenberger MA, Greenberg RE, Herr HW, Inman BA, Kuban DA, Kuzel TM, Lele SM, Michalski J, Pagliaro LC, Pal SK, Patterson A, Plimack ER, Pohar KS, Porter MP, Richie JP, Sexton WJ, Shipley WU, Small EJ, Spiess PE, Trump DL, Wile G, Wilson TG, Dwyer M, Ho M, National Comprehensive Cancer N. Bladder cancer. J Nat Compr Cancer Network JNCCN. 2013;11(4):446–75.
7. Hall MC, Chang SS, Dalbagni G, Pruthi R, Schellhammer PF, Seigne JD, Skinner E, Wolf JS, Jr. AUA Guideline for the management of nonmuscle invasive bladder cancer (stages Ta, T1, and Tis): 2007 Update; 2007. www.auanet.org/education/guidelines/bladder-cancer.cfm.Accessed 5/28/2015
8. Herranz-Amo F, Diez-Cordero JM, Verdu-Tartajo F, Bueno-Chomon G, Leal-Hernandez F, Bielsa-Carrillo A. Need for intravenous urography in patients with primary transitional carcinoma of the bladder? Eur Urol. 1999;36(3):221–4. doi:68001.
9. Palou J, Rodriguez-Rubio F, Huguet J, Segarra J, Ribal MJ, Alcaraz A, Villavicencio H. Multivariate analysis of clinical parameters of synchronous primary superficial bladder cancer and upper urinary tract tumor. J Urol. 2005;174(3):859–61. doi:10.1097/01.ju.0000169424.79702.6d. discussion 861.
10. Solsona E, Iborra I, Ricos JV, Dumont R, Casanova JL, Calabuig C. Upper urinary tract involvement in patients with bladder carcinoma in situ (Tis): its impact on management. Urology. 1997;49(3):347–52. doi:10.1016/S0090-4295(96)00571-7.
11. Holmang S, Hedelin H, Anderstrom C, Johansson SL. The relationship among multiple recurrences, progression and prognosis of patients with stages Ta and T1 transitional cell cancer of the bladder followed for at least 20 years. J Urol. 1995;153(6):1823–6. discussion 1826–1827.
12. Herr HW. Extravesical tumor relapse in patients with superficial bladder tumors. J Clin Oncol Off J Am Soc Clin Oncol. 1998;16(3):1099–102.
13. Hurle R, Losa A, Manzetti A, Lembo A. Upper urinary tract tumors developing after treatment of superficial bladder cancer: 7-year follow-up of 591 consecutive patients. Urology. 1999;53(6):1144–8.
14. Millan-Rodriguez F, Chechile-Toniolo G, Salvador-Bayarri J, Huguet-Perez J, Vicente-Rodriguez J. Upper urinary tract tumors after primary superficial bladder tumors: prognostic factors and risk groups. J Urol. 2000;164(4):1183–7.
15. Canales BK, Anderson JK, Premoli J, Slaton JW. Risk factors for upper tract recurrence in patients undergoing long-term surveillance for stage ta bladder cancer. J Urol. 2006;175(1):74–7. doi:10.1016/S0022-5347(05)00071-6.
16. Sternberg IA, Keren Paz GE, Chen LY, Herr HW, Donat SM, Bochner BH, Dalbagni G. Upper tract imaging surveillance is not effective in diagnosing upper tract recurrence in patients followed for nonmuscle invasive bladder cancer. J Urol. 2013;190(4):1187–91. doi:10.1016/j.juro.2013.05.020.
17. Amar AD, Das S. Upper urinary tract transitional cell carcinoma in patients with bladder carcinoma and associated vesicoureteral reflux. J Urol. 1985;133(3):468–71.
18. De Torres Mateos JA, Banus Gassol JM, Palou Redorta J, Morote Robles J. Vesicorenal reflux and upper urinary tract transitional cell carcinoma after transurethral resection of recurrence superficial bladder carcinoma. J Urol. 1987;138:49–51.
19. Shinka T, Uekado Y, Aoshi H, Hirano A, Ohkawa T. Occurrence of uroepithelial tumors of the upper urinary tract after the initial diagnosis of bladder cancer. J Urol. 1988;140(4):745–8.
20. Wright JL, Hotaling J, Porter MP. Predictors of upper tract urothelial cell carcinoma after primary bladder cancer: a population based analysis. J Urol. 2009;181(3):1035–9. doi:10.1016/j.juro.2008.10.168. discussion 1039.

21. Soukup V, Babjuk M, Bellmunt J, Dalbagni G, Giannarini G, Hakenberg OW, Herr H, Lechevallier E, Ribal MJ. Follow-up after surgical treatment of bladder cancer: a critical analysis of the literature. Eur Urol. 2012;62(2):290–302. doi:10.1016/j.eururo.2012.05.008.

22. Rabbani F, Perrotti M, Russo P, Herr HW. Upper-tract tumors after an initial diagnosis of bladder cancer: argument for long-term surveillance. J Clin Oncol Off J Am Soc Clin Oncol. 2001;19(1):94–100.

23. Learner SP, Sternberg CN. Chapter 82. Management of metastatic and invasive bladder cancer. In: Wein AJ, Kavoussi LR, Campbell MF, editors. Campbell-Walsh urology. 10th ed. Philadelphia: Elsevier Saunders; 2012.

24. Solsona E, Iborra I, Rubio J, Casanova J, Dumont R, Monros JL. Late oncological occurrences following radical cystectomy in patients with bladder cancer. Eur Urol. 2003;43(5):489–94.

25. Umbreit EC, Crispen PL, Shimko MS, Farmer SA, Blute ML, Frank I. Multifactorial, site-specific recurrence model after radical cystectomy for urothelial carcinoma. Cancer. 2010;116(14):3399–407. doi:10.1002/cncr.25202.

26. Balaji KC, McGuire M, Grotas J, Grimaldi G, Russo P. Upper tract recurrences following radical cystectomy: an analysis of prognostic factors, recurrence pattern and stage at presentation. J Urol. 1999;162(5):1603–6.

27. Furukawa J, Miyake H, Hara I, Takenaka A, Fujisawa M. Upper urinary tract recurrence following radical cystectomy for bladder cancer. Int J Urol Off J Jpn Urol Assoc. 2007;14(6):496–9. doi:10.1111/j.1442-2042.2007.01776.x.

28. Kenworthy P, Tanguay S, Dinney CP. The risk of upper tract recurrence following cystectomy in patients with transitional cell carcinoma involving the distal ureter. J Urol. 1996;155(2):501–3.

29. Sanderson KM, Cai J, Miranda G, Skinner DG, Stein JP. Upper tract urothelial recurrence following radical cystectomy for transitional cell carcinoma of the bladder: an analysis of 1,069 patients with 10-year followup. J Urol. 2007;177(6):2088–94. doi:10.1016/j.juro.2007.01.133.

30. Sved PD, Gomez P, Nieder AM, Manoharan M, Kim SS, Soloway MS. Upper tract tumour after radical cystectomy for transitional cell carcinoma of the bladder: incidence and risk factors. BJU Int. 2004;94(6):785–9. doi:10.1111/j.1464-410X.2004.05032.x.

31. Takayanagi A, Masumori N, Takahashi A, Takagi Y, Tsukamoto T. Upper urinary tract recurrence after radical cystectomy for bladder cancer: incidence and risk factors. Int J Urol Off J Jpn Urol Assoc. 2012;19(3):229–33. doi:10.1111/j.1442-2042.2011.02916.x.

32. Tran W, Serio AM, Raj GV, Dalbagni G, Vickers AJ, Bochner BH, Herr H, Donat SM. Longitudinal risk of upper tract recurrence following radical cystectomy for urothelial cancer and the potential implications for long-term surveillance. J Urol. 2008;179(1):96–100. doi:10.1016/j.juro.2007.08.131.

33. Volkmer BG, Schnoeller T, Kuefer R, Gust K, Finter F, Hautmann RE. Upper urinary tract recurrence after radical cystectomy for bladder cancer–who is at risk? J Urol. 2009;182(6):2632–7. doi:10.1016/j.juro.2009.08.046.

34. Perlis N, Turker P, Bostrom PJ, Kuk C, Mirtti T, Kulkarni G, Fleshner NE, Jewett MA, Finelli A, Zlotta AR. Upper urinary tract and urethral recurrences following radical cystectomy: review of risk factors and outcomes between centres with different follow-up protocols. World J Urol. 2013;31(1):161–7. doi:10.1007/s00345-012-0905-2.

35. Picozzi S, Ricci C, Gaeta M, Ratti D, Macchi A, Casellato S, Bozzini G, Carmignani L. Upper urinary tract recurrence following radical cystectomy for bladder cancer: a meta-analysis on 13,185 patients. J Urol. 2012;188(6):2046–54. doi:10.1016/j.juro.2012.08.017.

36. Stein JP. Should frozen section examination of the ureteral margins be routinely performed during cystectomy? Nat Clin Pract Urol. 2007;4(10):536–7. doi:10.1038/ncpuro0914.

37. Raj GV, Tal R, Vickers A, Bochner BH, Serio A, Donat SM, Herr H, Olgac S, Dalbagni G. Significance of intraoperative ureteral evaluation at radical cystectomy for urothelial cancer. Cancer. 2006;107(9):2167–72. doi:10.1002/cncr.22238.

38. Schumacher MC, Scholz M, Weise ES, Fleischmann A, Thalmann GN, Studer UE. Is there an indication for frozen section examination of the ureteral margins during cystectomy for transitional cell carcinoma of the bladder? J Urol. 2006;176(6 Pt 1):2409–13. doi:10.1016/j.juro.2006.07.162. discussion 2413.

39. Tollefson MK, Blute ML, Farmer SA, Frank I. Significance of distal ureteral margin at radical cystectomy for urothelial carcinoma. J Urol. 2010;183(1):81–6. doi:10.1016/j.juro.2009.08.158.

40. Donat SM. Argument against frozen section analysis of distal ureters in transitional cell bladder cancer. Nat Clin Pract Urol. 2008;5(10):538–9. doi:10.1038/ncpuro1210.

41. Meissner C, Giannarini G, Schumacher MC, Thoeny H, Studer UE, Burkhard FC. The efficiency of excretory urography to detect upper urinary tract tumors after cystectomy for urothelial cancer. J Urol. 2007;178(6):2287–90. doi:10.1016/j.juro.2007.08.041.

42. Boorjian SA, Tollefson MK, Cheville JC, Costello BA, Thapa P, Frank I. Detection of asymptomatic recurrence during routine oncological followup after radical cystectomy is associated with improved patient survival. J Urol. 2011;186(5):1796–802. doi:10.1016/j.juro.2011.07.005.

43. Fernandez MI, Parikh S, Grossman HB, Katz R, Matin SF, Dinney CP, Kamat AM. The role of FISH and cytology in upper urinary tract surveillance after radical cystectomy for bladder cancer. Urol Oncol. 2012;30(6):821–4. doi:10.1016/j.urolonc.2010.08.006.

44. Shinagare AB, Sadow CA, Silverman SG. Surveillance of patients with bladder cancer following cystectomy: yield of CT urography.

Abdom Imaging. 2013;38(6):1415–21. doi:10.1007/s00261-013-0024-6.

45. Pieras E, Frontera G, Ruiz X, Vicens A, Ozonas M, Piza P. Concomitant carcinoma in situ and tumour size are prognostic factors for bladder recurrence after nephroureterectomy for upper tract transitional cell carcinoma. BJU Int. 2010;106(9):1319–23. doi:10.1111/j.1464-410X.2010.09341.x.

46. Matsui Y, Utsunomiya N, Ichioka K, Ueda N, Yoshimura K, Terai A, Arai Y. Risk factors for subsequent development of bladder cancer after primary transitional cell carcinoma of the upper urinary tract. Urology. 2005;65(2):279–83. doi:10.1016/j.urology.2004.09.021.

47. Xylinas E, Rink M, Cha EK, Clozel T, Lee RK, Fajkovic H, Comploj E, Novara G, Margulis V, Raman JD, Lotan Y, Kassouf W, Fritsche HM, Weizer A, Martinez-Salamanca JI, Matsumoto K, Zigeuner R, Pycha A, Scherr DS, Seitz C, Walton T, Trinh QD, Karakiewicz PI, Matin S, Montorsi F, Zerbib M, Shariat SF, Upper Tract Urothelial Carcinoma Collaboration. Impact of distal ureter management on oncologic outcomes following radical nephroureterectomy for upper tract urothelial carcinoma. Eur Urol. 2014;65(1):210–7. doi:10.1016/j.eururo.2012.04.052.

48. Hisataki T, Miyao N, Masumori N, Takahashi A, Sasai M, Yanase M, Itoh N, Tsukamoto T. Risk factors for the development of bladder cancer after upper tract urothelial cancer. Urology. 2000;55(5):663–7.

49. Zigeuner RE, Hutterer G, Chromecki T, Rehak P, Langner C. Bladder tumour development after urothelial carcinoma of the upper urinary tract is related to primary tumour location. BJU Int. 2006;98(6):1181–6. doi:10.1111/j.1464-410X.2006.06519.x.

50. Mukamel E, Simon D, Edelman A, Konichezky M, Hadar H, Servadio C. Metachronous bladder tumors in patients with upper urinary tract transitional cell carcinoma. J Surg Oncol. 1994;57(3):187–90.

51. Koga F, Nagamatsu H, Ishimaru H, Mizuo T, Yoshida K. Risk factors for the development of bladder transitional cell carcinoma following surgery for transitional cell carcinoma of the upper urinary tract. Urol Int. 2001;67(2):135–41. doi:50969.

52. Li CC, Chang TH, Wu WJ, Ke HL, Huang SP, Tsai PC, Chang SJ, Shen JT, Chou YH, Huang CH. Significant predictive factors for prognosis of primary upper urinary tract cancer after radical nephroureterectomy in Taiwanese patients. Eur Urol. 2008;54(5):1127–34. doi:10.1016/j.eururo.2008.01.054.

53. Raman JD, Ng CK, Boorjian SA, Vaughan Jr ED, Sosa RE, Scherr DS. Bladder cancer after managing upper urinary tract transitional cell carcinoma: predictive factors and pathology. BJU Int. 2005;96(7):1031–5. doi:10.1111/j.1464-410X.2005.05804.x.

54. Novara G, De Marco V, Dalpiaz O, Gottardo F, Bouygues V, Galfano A, Martignoni G, Patard JJ, Artibani W, Ficarra V. Independent predictors of metachronous bladder transitional cell carcinoma (TCC) after nephroureterectomy for TCC of the upper urinary tract. BJU Int. 2008;101(11):1368–74. doi:10.1111/j.1464-410X.2008.07438.x.

55. Xylinas E, Colin P, Audenet F, Phe V, Cormier L, Cussenot O, Houlgatte A, Karsenty G, Bruyere F, Polguer T, Ruffion A, Valeri A, Rozet F, Long JA, Zerbib M, Roupret M. Intravesical recurrence after radical nephroureterectomy for upper tract urothelial carcinomas: predictors and impact on subsequent oncological outcomes from a national multicenter study. World J Urol. 2013;31(1):61–8. doi:10.1007/s00345-012-0957-3.

56. Walton TJ, Novara G, Matsumoto K, Kassouf W, Fritsche HM, Artibani W, Bastian PJ, Martinez-Salamanca JI, Seitz C, Thomas SA, Ficarra V, Burger M, Tritschler S, Karakiewicz PI, Shariat SF. Oncological outcomes after laparoscopic and open radical nephroureterectomy: results from an international cohort. BJU Int. 2011;108(3):406–12. doi:10.1111/j.1464-410X.2010.09826.x.

57. Capitanio U, Shariat SF, Isbarn H, Weizer A, Remzi M, Roscigno M, Kikuchi E, Raman JD, Bolenz C, Bensalah K, Koppie TM, Kassouf W, Fernandez MI, Strobel P, Wheat J, Zigeuner R, Langner C, Waldert M, Oya M, Guo CC, Ng C, Montorsi F, Wood CG, Margulis V, Karakiewicz PI. Comparison of oncologic outcomes for open and laparoscopic nephroureterectomy: a multi-institutional analysis of 1249 cases. Eur Urol. 2009;56(1):1–9. doi:10.1016/j.eururo.2009.03.072.

58. Favaretto RL, Shariat SF, Chade DC, Godoy G, Kaag M, Cronin AM, Bochner BH, Coleman J, Dalbagni G. Comparison between laparoscopic and open radical nephroureterectomy in a contemporary group of patients: are recurrence and disease-specific survival associated with surgical technique? Eur Urol. 2010;58(5):645–51. doi:10.1016/j.eururo.2010.08.005.

59. Krogh J, Kvist E, Rye B. Transitional cell carcinoma of the upper urinary tract: prognostic variables and postoperative recurrences. Br J Urol. 1991;67(1):32–6.

60. Roupret M, Babjuk M, Comperat E, Zigeuner R, Sylvester R, Burger M, Cowan N, Bohle A, Van Rhijn BW, Kaasinen E, Palou J, Shariat SF, European Association of Urology. European guidelines on upper tract urothelial carcinomas: 2013 update. Eur Urol. 2013;63(6):1059–71. doi:10.1016/j.eururo.2013.03.032.

61. Salvador-Bayarri J, Rodriguez-Villamil L, Imperatore V, Palou Redorta J, Villavicencio-Mavrich H, Vicente-Rodriguez J. Bladder neoplasms after nephroureterectomy: does the surgery of the lower ureter, transurethral resection or open surgery, influence the evolution? Eur Urol. 2002;41(1):30–3.

62. Chen MK, Ye YL, Zhou FJ, Liu JY, Lu KS, Han H, Liu ZW, Xu ZZ, Qin ZK. Clipping the extremity of ureter prior to nephroureterectomy is effective in preventing subsequent bladder recurrence after upper urinary tract urothelial carcinoma. Chin Med J (Engl). 2012;125(21):3821–6.

63. Tolley DA, Parmar MK, Grigor KM, Lallemand G, Benyon LL, Fellows J, Freedman LS, Grigor KM, Hall RR, Hargreave TB, Munson K, Newling DW, Richards B, Robinson MR, Rose MB, Smith PH, Williams JL, Whelan P. The effect of intravesical mitomycin C on recurrence of newly diagnosed

superficial bladder cancer: a further report with 7 years of follow up. J Urol. 1996;155(4):1233–8.

64. Oosterlinck W, Kurth KH, Schroder F, Bultinck J, Hammond B, Sylvester R. A prospective European Organization for Research and Treatment of Cancer Genitourinary Group randomized trial comparing transurethral resection followed by a single intravesical instillation of epirubicin or water in single stage Ta, T1 papillary carcinoma of the bladder. J Urol. 1993;149(4):749–52.

65. Bouffioux C, Kurth KH, Bono A, Oosterlinck W, Kruger CB, De Pauw M, Sylvester R. Intravesical adjuvant chemotherapy for superficial transitional cell bladder carcinoma: results of 2 European Organization for Research and Treatment of Cancer randomized trials with mitomycin C and doxorubicin comparing early versus delayed installations and short-term versus long-term treatment. European Organization for Research and Treatment of Cancer Genitourinary Group. J Urol. 1995;153(3 Pt 2):934–41.

66. Sakamoto N, Naito S, Kumazawa J, Ariyoshi A, Osada Y, Omoto T, Fujisawa Y, Morita I, Yamashita H, Kyushu University Urological Oncology Group. Prophylactic intravesical instillation of mitomycin C and cytosine arabinoside for prevention of recurrent bladder tumors following surgery for upper urinary tract tumors: a prospective randomized study. Int J Urol Off J Jpn Urol Assoc. 2001;8(5):212–6.

67. Ito A, Shintaku I, Satoh M, Ioritani N, Aizawa M, Tochigi T, Kawamura S, Aoki H, Numata I, Takeda A, Namiki S, Namima T, Ikeda Y, Kambe K, Kyan A, Ueno S, Orikasa K, Katoh S, Adachi H, Tokuyama S, Ishidoya S, Yamaguchi T, Arai Y. Prospective randomized phase II trial of a single early intravesical instillation of pirarubicin (THP) in the prevention of bladder recurrence after nephroureterectomy for upper urinary tract urothelial carcinoma: the THP Monotherapy Study Group Trial. J Clin Oncol Off J Am Soc Clin Oncol. 2013;31(11):1422 7. doi:10.1200/JCO.2012.45.2128.

68. Mullerad M, Russo P, Golijanin D, Chen HN, Tsai HH, Donat SM, Bochner BH, Herr HW, Sheinfeld J, Sogani PC, Kattan MW, Dalbagni G. Bladder cancer as a prognostic factor for upper tract transitional cell carcinoma. J Urol. 2004;172(6 Pt 1):2177–81.

69. Colin P, Koenig P, Ouzzane A, Berthon N, Villers A, Biserte J, Roupret M. Environmental factors involved in carcinogenesis of urothelial cell carcinomas of the upper urinary tract. BJU Int. 2009;104(10):1436–40. doi:10.1111/j.1464-410X.2009.08838.x.

70. Laing C, Hamour S, Sheaff M, Miller R, Woolfson R. Chinese herbal uropathy and nephropathy. Lancet. 2006;368(9532):338. doi:10.1016/S0140-6736(06)69079-X.

71. Nortier JL, Martinez MC, Schmeiser HH, Arlt VM, Bieler CA, Petein M, Depierreux MF, De Pauw L, Abramowicz D, Vereerstraeten P, Vanherweghem JL. Urothelial carcinoma associated with the use of a Chinese herb (Aristolochia fangchi). N Engl J Med. 2000;342(23):1686–92. doi:10.1056/NEJM200006083422301.

72. Sijmons RH, Kiemeney LA, Witjes JA, Vasen HF. Urinary tract cancer and hereditary nonpolyposis colorectal cancer: risks and screening options. J Urol. 1998;160(2):466–70.

73. Roupret M, Yates DR, Comperat E, Cussenot O. Upper urinary tract urothelial cell carcinomas and other urological malignancies involved in the hereditary nonpolyposis colorectal cancer (lynch syndrome) tumor spectrum. Eur Urol. 2008;54(6):1226–36. doi:10.1016/j.eururo.2008.08.008.

74. Skeldon SC, Semotiuk K, Aronson M, Holter S, Gallinger S, Pollett A, Kuk C, van Rhijn B, Bostrom P, Cohen Z, Fleshner NE, Jewett MA, Hanna S, Shariat SF, Van Der Kwast TH, Evans A, Catto J, Bapat B, Zlotta AR. Patients with Lynch syndrome mismatch repair gene mutations are at higher risk for not only upper tract urothelial cancer but also bladder cancer. Eur Urol. 2013;63(2):379–85. doi:10.1016/j.eururo.2012.07.047.

75. Catto JW, Azzouzi AR, Rehman I, Feeley KM, Cross SS, Amira N, Fromont G, Sibony M, Cussenot O, Meuth M, Hamdy FC. Promoter hypermethylation is associated with tumor location, stage, and subsequent progression in transitional cell carcinoma. J Clin Oncol Off J Am Soc Clin Oncol. 2005;23(13):2903–10. doi:10.1200/JCO.2005.03.163.

76. Mao L, Lee DJ, Tockman MS, Erozan YS, Askin F, Sidransky D. Microsatellite alterations as clonal markers for the detection of human cancer. Proc Natl Acad Sci U S A. 1994;91(21):9871–5.

77. Danaee H, Nelson HH, Karagas MR, Schned AR, Ashok TD, Hirao T, Perry AE, Kelsey KT. Microsatellite instability at tetranucleotide repeats in skin and bladder cancer. Oncogene. 2002;21(32):4894–9. doi:10.1038/sj.onc.1205619.

78. Catto JW, Azzouzi AR, Amira N, Rehman I, Feeley KM, Cross SS, Fromont G, Sibony M, Hamdy FC, Cussenot O, Meuth M. Distinct patterns of microsatellite instability are seen in tumours of the urinary tract. Oncogene. 2003;22(54):8699–706. doi:10.1038/sj.onc.1206964.

79. Rigola MA, Fuster C, Casadevall C, Bernues M, Caballin MR, Gelabert A, Egozcue J, Miro R. Comparative genomic hybridization analysis of transitional cell carcinomas of the renal pelvis. Cancer Genet Cytogenet. 2001;127(1):59–63.

80. Czerniak B, Chaturvedi V, Li L, Hodges S, Johnston D, Roy JY, Luthra R, Logothetis C, Von Eschenbach AC, Grossman HB, Benedict WF, Batsakis JG. Superimposed histologic and genetic mapping of chromosome 9 in progression of human urinary bladder neoplasia: implications for a genetic model of multistep urothelial carcinogenesis and early detection of urinary bladder cancer. Oncogene. 1999;18(5):1185–96. doi:10.1038/sj.onc.1202385.

81. Hoglund M, Sall T, Heim S, Mitelman F, Mandahl N, Fadl-Elmula I. Identification of cytogenetic subgroups and karyotypic pathways in transitional cell carcinoma. Cancer Res. 2001;61(22):8241–6.

82. Hurst CD, Fiegler H, Carr P, Williams S, Carter NP, Knowles MA. High-resolution analysis of genomic copy number alterations in bladder cancer by microarray-based comparative genomic hybridization. Oncogene. 2004;23(12):2250–63. doi:10.1038/sj.onc.1207260.

83. Veltman JA, Fridlyand J, Pejavar S, Olshen AB, Korkola JE, DeVries S, Carroll P, Kuo WL, Pinkel D, Albertson D, Cordon-Cardo C, Jain AN, Waldman FM. Array-based comparative genomic hybridization for genome-wide screening of DNA copy number in bladder tumors. Cancer Res. 2003;63(11):2872–80.

84. Akao J, Matsuyama H, Yamamoto Y, Sasaki K, Naito K. Chromosome 20q13.2 gain may predict intravesical recurrence after nephroureterectomy in upper urinary tract urothelial tumors. Clin Cancer Res Off J Am Assoc Cancer Res. 2006;12(23):7004–8. doi:10.1158/1078-0432.CCR-06-0825.

85. van Oers JM, Zwarthoff EC, Rehman I, Azzouzi AR, Cussenot O, Meuth M, Hamdy FC, Catto JW. FGFR3 mutations indicate better survival in invasive upper urinary tract and bladder tumours. Eur Urol. 2009;55(3):650–7. doi:10.1016/j.eururo.2008.06.013.

86. Izquierdo L, Mengual L, Gazquez C, Ingelmo-Torres M, Alcaraz A. Molecular characterization of upper urinary tract tumours. BJU Int. 2010;106(6):868–72. doi:10.1111/j.1464-410X.2009.09135.x.

87. Zhang Z, Furge KA, Yang XJ, Teh BT, Hansel DE. Comparative gene expression profiling analysis of urothelial carcinoma of the renal pelvis and bladder. BMC Med Genomics. 2010;3:58. doi:10.1186/1755-8794-3-58.

88. Jones JS, Larchian W. Chapter 81. Non-muscle-invasive bladder cancer (Ta, T1, and CIS). In: Campbell-Walsh urology. 10th ed. Philadelphia: W.B. Saunders Co.; 2012.

89. Sakamoto N, Naito S, Kotoh S, Nakashima M, Nakamura M, Ueda T, Kumazawa J. Recurrence of bladder tumors following surgery for transitional cell carcinoma of the upper urinary tract. Eur Urol. 1991;20(2):136–9.

90. Hall MC, Womack S, Sagalowsky AI, Carmody T, Erickstad MD, Roehrborn CG. Prognostic factors, recurrence, and survival in transitional cell carcinoma of the upper urinary tract: a 30-year experience in 252 patients. Urology. 1998;52(4):594–601.

Enhanced Imaging: NBI, PDD, SPIES

11

Luca Villa, Jonathan Cloutier, and Olivier Traxer

Over the last decade, minimally-invasive surgery has gained popularity in the urological field as a valid treatment option for the conservative management of upper urinary tract transitional cell carcinoma (UUT-TCC).

In this context, flexible ureteroscopy represents an ideal solution. Indeed, it allows the urologist to complete the diagnostic process as well as to offer a curative treatment, performing a complete visual inspection of the renal collecting system and using holmium-YAG laser for tumour photoablation, respectively.

However, several aspects still need to be improved for optimising the endoscopic treatment of UUT-TCC. The major concern is the quality of view, which is strictly connected with the imaging system characterizing the ureteroscope adopted for the procedure and this is crucial for the outcome of the procedure. The introduction of digital ureteroscopes from different companies has guaranteed a definitive improvement of the quality of view with regard to the images obtained with fiber optic ureteroscope [1, 2], and this is particularly important when aiming at diagnosing and conservatively treating UUT-TCC, especially in presence of small and/or flat tumour which could be difficult to be identified (see Fig. 11.1).

Moreover, an adequate staging of UUT-TCC patients can be hampered by technical difficulties in obtaining reliable pathological data with the ureteroscopic biopsy [3, 4]. Finally, not all the urothelial malignant lesions are always visible using white light, which represents the standard source of light of the standard endourological procedures. In the field of bladder cancer, enhanced imaging techniques are being developed with the aim of increase the diagnostic accuracy of cystocopy and improve the outocome of transurethral resection of the bladder (TURB) [5]. Nevertheless, these new technologies are being applied to the endoscopic management of malignancies of the upper urinary tract, with promising results.

In this chapter we sought to describe the different enhanced imaging techniques available on the market and the preliminary results of these devices when applied to the treatment of UUT-TCC.

L. Villa, MD
Department of Urology, Tenon University Hospital, Hôpitaux de Paris, Pierre et Marie Curie University, 4 rue de la Chine, Paris 75020, France

Department of Urology, Universita Vita-Salute San Raffaele, San Raffaele Hospital, Via Olgettina 60, Milan 20132, Italy
e-mail: l.villa@hotmail.it

J. Cloutier, MD, FRCSC • O. Traxer, MD, PhD (✉)
Department of Urology, Tenon University Hospital, Hôpitaux de Paris, Pierre et Marie Curie University, 4 rue de la Chine, Paris 75020, France
e-mail: Jonathan.cloutier.2@ulaval.ca; Olivier.traxer@tnn.aphp.fr

© Springer International Publishing Switzerland 2015
M. Grasso III, D.H. Bagley (eds.), *Upper Urinary Tract Urothelial Carcinoma,*
DOI 10.1007/978-3-319-13869-5_11

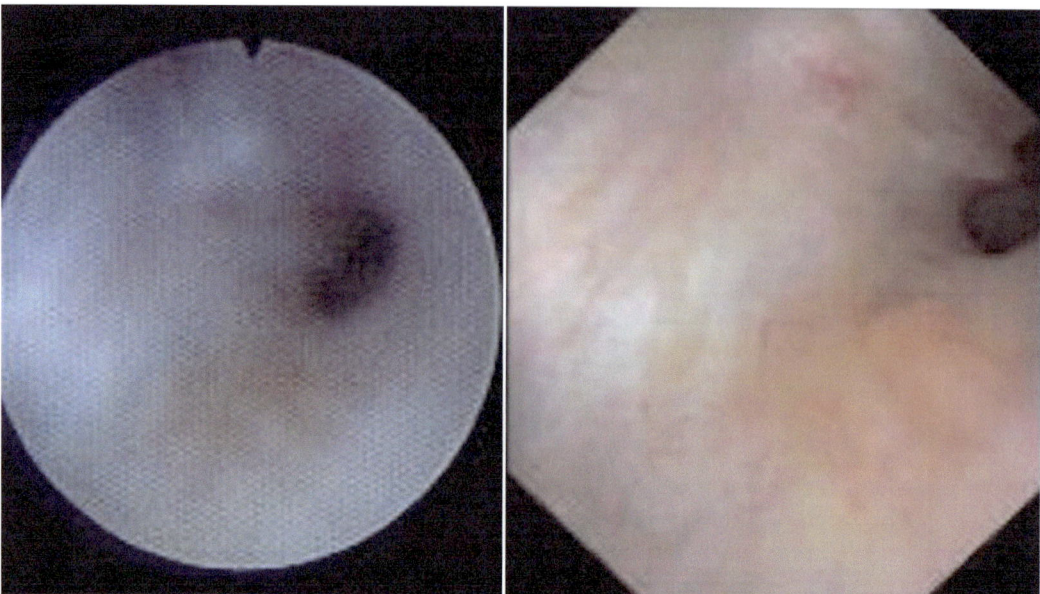

Fig. 11.1 Endoscopic view of a superficial urothelial lesion of the left renal pelvis with a fiber optic (*left*) and a digital (*right*) ureteroscope

11.1 Narrow Band Imaging (NBI)

Narrow Band Imaging (NBI) system has been incorporated by Olympus in the endoscopic instrumentation. It consists of a new function for detecting suspicious lesions in the urinary tract which adopts the FWL system, an optical image technology that enhances the contrast between normal urothelium and cancer tissue by filtering white light into two bandwidths of 415 and 540 nm. These narrow bands of light are strongly absorbed by haemoglobin and penetrate the tissue surface only, increasing the visibility of mucosal vascular structures. As result, capillaries are displayed in brown and veins in the sub-surface are displayed in cyan on the operating monitor [6] (see Fig. 11.2).

Due to the vascular nature of urothelial carcinoma, NBI enhances the contrast between superficial tumours and normal mucosa. Subjectively, NBI clearly shows the specific vascular architecture of UUT-TCC, creating the impression of a 3D visualisation of the malignant lesion and improving the definition of tumour edges.

Therefore, the spatial representation of tumours may affect the diagnostic accuracy of the endoscopic procedure, thus increasing the detection of all those malignant lesions not perfectly visible with white light.

This in turn may lead to improve the likelihood of complete tumour ablation, absence of tumour persistence at the end of the procedure and to reduce the risk of tumour recurrence. Data available in literature showed that cancer detection rate in patients undergoing NBI cystoscopy was higher than that of their white light cystoscopy counterparts [7]. Moreover, NBI cystoscopy performed after white light cystoscopy increased the detection of malignant lesions by 13–41 % [8, 9].

Finally, NBI has been proven to have a positive impact on the risk of tumour recurrence at 1 year after initial TURB. Indeed, it has been reported at 32.9 % in the NBI group versus 51.4 % in the white light group [10].

11.1.1 Incorporation in Video-Ureteroscopy

NBI system has been recently incorporated by Olympus in the digital ureteroscopes (namely, URF-V and URF-V2). As described in the field of bladder cancer, the current technique is expected

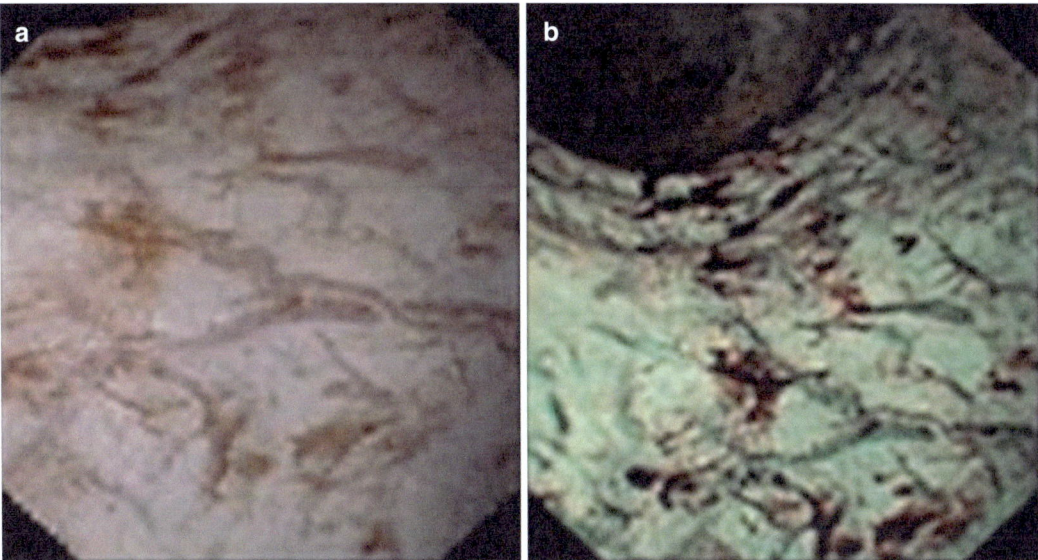

Fig. 11.2 Normal urothelium. (**a**) Endoscopic view with white-light cystoscopy; (**b**) Narrow-band imaging cystoscopy

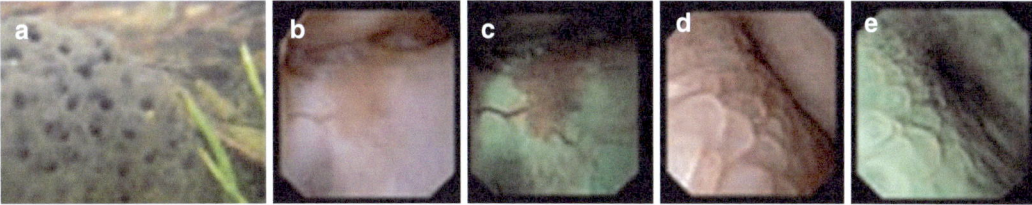

Fig. 11.3 (**a**) Frog's eggs; (**b**) Urothelial tumour with white-light ureterorenoscopy; (**c**) Urothelial tumour with narrow-band imaging system 'frog's eggs effect'; (**d**) Urothelial irritation due to JJ stent (white-light ureterorenoscopy); and (**e**) Urothelial irritation due to JJ stent (narrow-band imaging system) with no 'frog's eggs effect'

to help clinicians in the diagnosis of early urothelial carcinoma and particular condition, such as carcinoma in situ. Indeed, due to the microvascular component characterising malignant lesion, flat lesion can be clearly distinguished from edematous lesions caused for instances by JJ stent, appearing as "frog's eggs" (see Fig. 11.3).

11.1.2 Preliminary Results of NBI Technology in the Diagnosis of UUT-TCC

The first report regarding the use of such a technique in the field of endoscopic treatment of UUT-TCC came from Tenon University Hospital's experience. Data coming from 27 patients were analyzed. Any area in the NBI mode which appeared as discordant by either blood vessel concentration or appearance (i.e., dotted, tortuous, large-calibre, abrupt-ending vessels) as compared to white-light mode was considered as an abnormal appearance suspected of being malignant lesion. NBI technology allowed to diagnose and clearly visualise UUT-TCC and to identify the extended tumour limits (see Fig. 11.4).

When comparing the endoscopic results with bioptic findings, there were 35 pathologically confirmed transitional cell tumours detected. NBI diagnosed five tumours missed at WL (14.2 %) and clearly identified the edges of three

Fig. 11.4 Examples of endoscopic views with narrow band inaging (NBI) (*left*) and white-light (WL) (*right*). (**a**) Multiple lesion in pyelo-caliceal left kidney. (**b**) small lesion more visible with NBI versus WL. (**c**) Extent limits better identified with NBI versus WL. (**d**) No tumour visible in WL. Papillary tumour detected at NBI

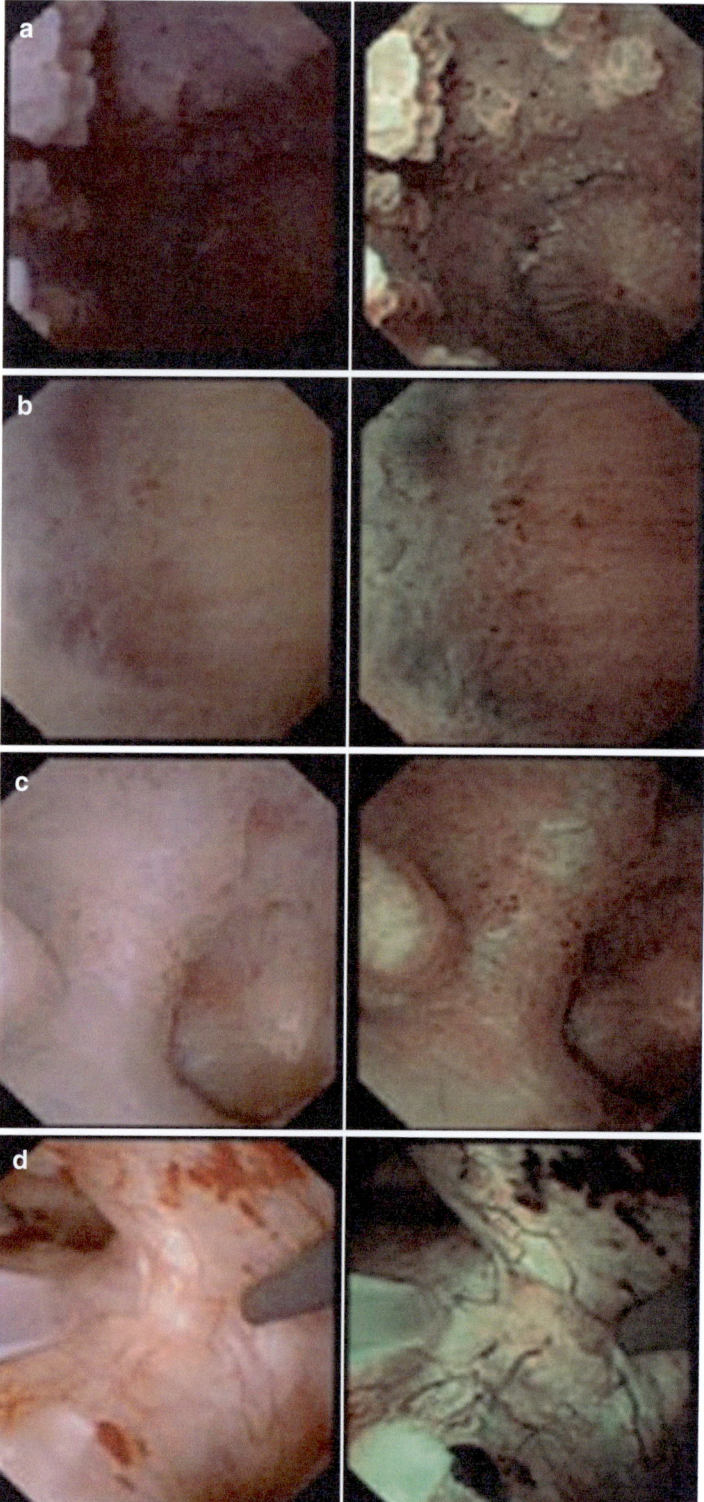

tumours (8.5 %), improving tumour detection rate by 22.7 % [11].

However, no specimens were taken from the extended margins of the tumours that were only visible by NBI, therefore the authors were not able to confirm the hypothesis that such a technique helps clinicians to discriminate tumour limits.

Taken together, these preliminary findings may be the basis for developing further studies aimed at confirming the benefit of NBI not only in the diagnosis but also in the long term treatment of UUT-TCC. Indeed, the impact of NBI technology on the risk of tumour recurrence and progression over time in these patients has still to be determined.

11.2 Photodynamic Diagnosis (PDD)

Photodynamic diagnosis (PDD) relies on fluorescence produced by substances with particular properties called fluorochromes which can be localized into abnormal tissue. This technique, initially employed for the diagnosis of other malignancies, such as lung cancer, skin cancer, upper aerodigestive tract cancer, has been increasingly used in the urological field to identify urothelial malignant lesions. PDD is able to improve the diagnosis of all those tumours which would not be clearly seen with standard endoscopic procedure due to their flat shape and/or small size [12].

The fluorescence occurs when the outer electrons of the fluorochrome return at their own ground state after having been excited by the absorption of a photon of appropriate wavelength. This technique has been designed as a combination of a photosensitizing drug, delivered orally or topically and spontaneously absorbed by abnormal cells, and a specific instrumentation equipped with a source of light able to excite the substance itself by using specific wavelengths, thus enhancing specific fluorescence staining, and optical filters able to detect the fluorescent signal.

Among the substances available for PDD in the urological field, 5-aminolevulinic acid (5-ALA) is the most widely used.

11.2.1 5-ALA and Derivatives

5-ALA plays a natural role in the biosynthetic pathway of heme. Indeed, it is the metabolic precursor of protoporphyrin IX (PpIX), which is the only fluorescent substance in the pathway. The step from protoporphyrin IX (PpIX) to heme, which include the insertion of a ferrous ion into the porphyrin ring, is the critical bottleneck of the whole pathway. Therefore, an exogenous administration of 5-ALA will induce elevated intracellular level of PpIX and consequently an increased fluorescence staining activity arising from neoplastic or highly proliferating cells [13, 14]. This phenomenon has been used by clinicians to better identify malignant and premalignant lesions during endourological procedures. The fluorescent-mode light used is the blue light, which serves as a reference for the normal urothelium, while the tissue accumulating the compound appears as red (see Fig. 11.5).

Data available in literature showed that PDD increased the sensitivity of fluorescence-guided biopsy and resection compared to conventional procedure in the detection of urothelial bladder cancer, especially of carcinoma in situ (CIS), reduced the risk of residual tumour at the second resection and increased the recurrence free-survival [15, 16].

This diagnostic modality has been also tested in the upper urinary tract. In literature there is only one study describing the use of PDD in the management of UUT-TCC. In such a report, Omar et al. [17] performed diagnostic URS in 30 patients with suspicion of UU-TCC for positive cytology with negative findings or CT scan abnormalities, after having orally administered them 5-ALA 3–4 h before the procedure. All suspicious lesions were biopsied. Their findings showed that out of the 17 pathologically-confirmed malignant lesions, PDD-URS detected more UUT-TCC compared to white-light URS (WL-URS) and CT scan (94 % vs. 76.5 % vs. 82 %, respectively) and picked up the only three cases of CIS, which was not seen neither at WL-URS nor at CT scan. However, the sensitivity and specificity are reported as similar between the different procedures.

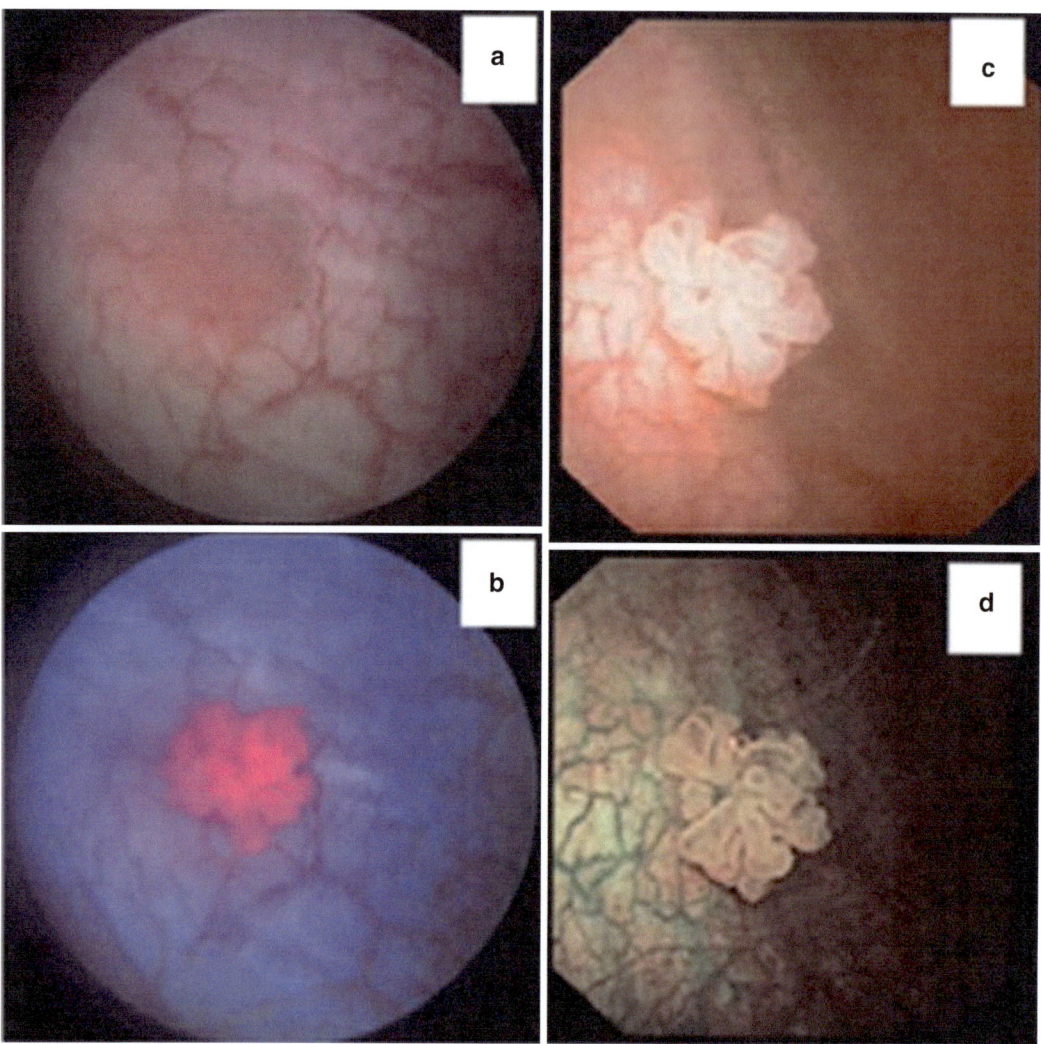

Fig. 11.5 Comparison of endoscopic visualization of a urothelial tumour with classic white-light (**a**), after 5-aminolevulanic acid instillation and blue light (**b**), with a white-light digital endoscope (**c**), and with NBI (**d**)

5-ALA may be also theoretically delivered by percutaneous nephrostomy or urinary stent, although the duration of exposure of the upper urinary tract mucosa to the compound might not be as long as necessary and the anatomy of the renal cavities might hamper an adequate flow of the compound into the whole intrarenal collecting system.

Unfortunately, the fluorescence signals arising from tissues are not as specific as in fluorescence microscopy, where the fluorochrome is bound to antibodies which selectively bind their target and can therefore be detected with high sensitivity.

Moreover, the detectable fluorescence staining from the fluorochrome is not a reliable quantitative measure of its local concentration [12].

Another major drawback of 5-ALA, which is transported intracellulary by an active uptake of membrane transport proteins, is represented by its low lipophilicity, thus reducing passive diffusion through the cell membrane. This is the main reason why ester derivatives of 5-ALA have been synthesised.

Such a compound, called Hexylester Hexaminolevulinate (developed by Photocure

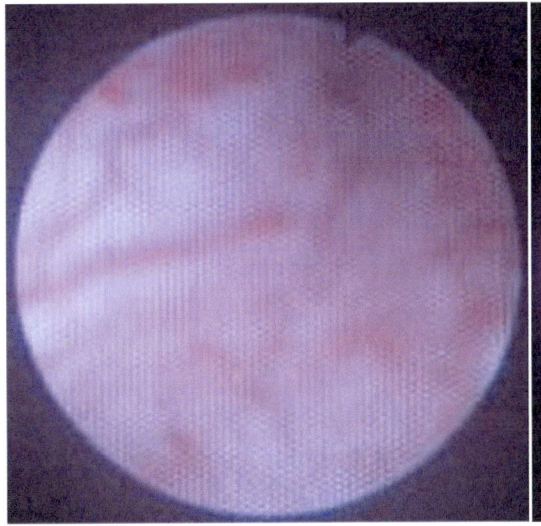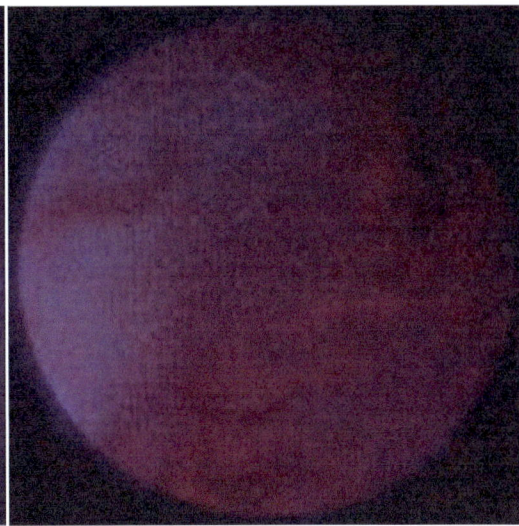

Fig. 11.6 Comparison of endoscopic visualization of a suspected urothelial tumour in the left renal pelvis with classic white-light (*left*) and after Hexvix® instillation and blue light (*right*) obtained with a fiber optic ureteroscope (Karl Storz PDD Flex-X2)

ASA, Norway and licensed by Ipsen as CysView® in US and Hexvix® in Europe) is characterized by a considerably faster and more efficient uptake, providing twice the fluorescence staining and requiring a half of the instillation time compared to 5-ALA (1 h vs. 2) [18]. However, it can be administered only topically by direct injection into the bladder, thus limiting its employment to the lower urinary tract only. In our personal experience we performed some cases of UUT-TCC with Hexvix® by delivering the compound into the renal cavities through a 7 Fr ureteral catheter. Due to the difficulties of properly releasing the drug in the area of interest and the lack of any digital ureteroscope incorporating an imaging system able to provide PDD, the quality of enhanced imaging obtained with a fiber optic ureteroscope (Karl Storz PDD Flex-X2) during such procedures was quite poor (see Fig. 11.6).

An alternative to the delivery of an exogenous compound that acts as a fluorochrome might be represented by the use of autofluorescence properties of various endogenous substances in the subepithelial connective tissue, for instances collagen and elastin. An abnormal proliferative activity usually results in an increased thickness of the epithelial layer, thus causing a reduction of the autofluorescence signal, which can be interpreted as an indirect sign of the presence of a malignant lesion [19, 20]. Although this technique may actually fit for the PDD of the UUT-TCC avoiding all the concerns related to the fluorochrome exogenous instillation, it has not yet been investigated in any clinical trial and it is not currently employed in the every-day clinical practice.

11.3 Storz Professional Imaging Enhancement System (SPIES)

Karl Storz company has recently developed a new system for enhanced imaging to be used in the field of endoscopic management of urothelial cancer.

This technology, called Storz Professional Image Enhancement System (SPIES®), allows to have an endoscopic view in four different modes, with two images on the screen (white-light image and enhanced image) without requiring any special light source.

In particular, SPECTRA modes (A and B) provide specific colour renderings that enhances local contrast related to the different penetration depth in the tissue.

Fig. 11.7 Comparison of endoscopic visualization of bladder urothelial tumour in white light (*left*) and Spectra A mode (*right*). (**a**) Pedunculated polyp of the upper left wall. (**b**) Sessile polyp of the posterior wall. (**c**) Superficial lesion of the posterior wall (By courtesy of Dr. G. Kamphuis and JJ de la Rosette)

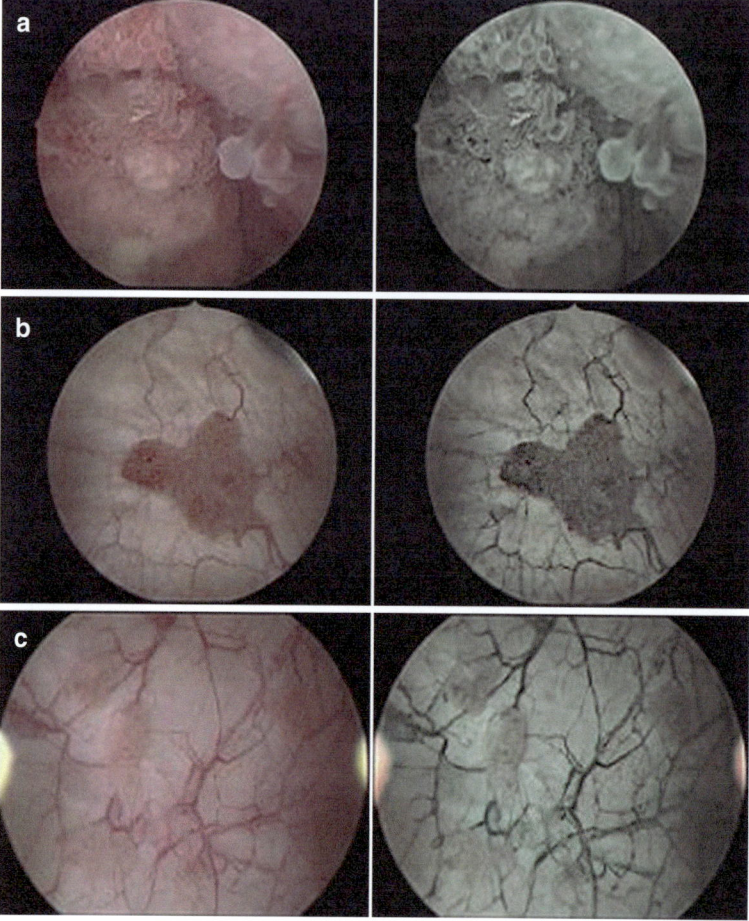

SPECTRA A is based on green and blue spectral signals. A colour transformation pronounces the contrasts within these spectral bands. Due to the short to mid-range tissue-penetration depth of the blue to green spectral part, this mode highlights the contrast of capillaries and vessels in (sub)mucosa (see Fig. 11.7).

On the other hand, SPECTRA B uses a colour tone algorithm to reduce the dominant diffuse red spectral reflection.

Similarly, contrast of capillaries and vessels in the (sub)mucosa are highlighted, without losing the additional information from deeper tissue layers that are only visible in the red spectral part (see Fig. 11.8).

A third mode (CLARA) provides clearer visibility of dark regions relying on local brightness adaptation thus enhancing light, while a fourth mode (CHROMA) enhances the sharpness of the anatomical structures displayed on the monitor by increasing colour contrast (see Fig. 11.9).

A clinical trial investigating the role of such a technique in the management of UUT-TCC is going to get started, and some preliminary cases have already been performed (see Fig. 11.10).

However, no data are currently available, therefore the effectiveness of SPIES in this field still need to be demonstrated.

Fig. 11.8 Comparison of endoscopic visualization of bladder urothelial tumour in white light (*left*) and combined Spectra B mode (*right*). (**a**) Pedunculated polyp of the upper left wall. (**b**) Sessile polyp of the posterior wall. (**c**) Superficial lesion of the posterior wall (By courtesy of Dr. G. Kamphuis and JJ de la Rosette)

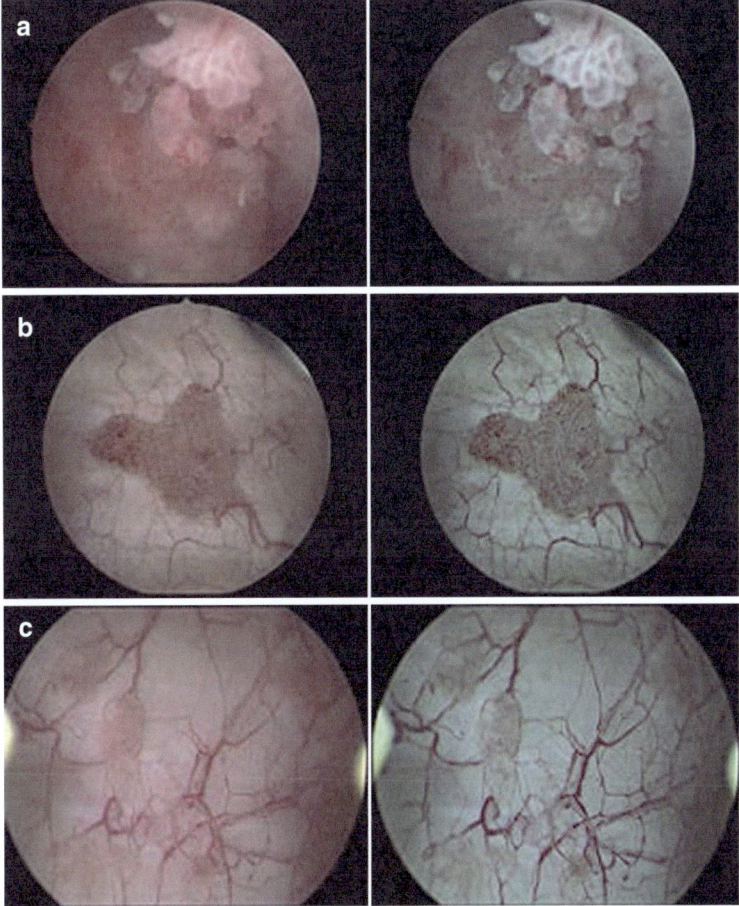

Fig. 11.9 Comparison of endoscopic visualization of bladder urothelial tumour in white light (*left*) and combined Chroma-Clara mode (*right*). (**a**) Pedunculated polyp of the upper left wall. (**b**) Sessile polyp of the posterior wall. (**c**) Superficial lesion of the posterior wall (By courtesy of Dr. G. Kamphuis and JJ de la Rosette)

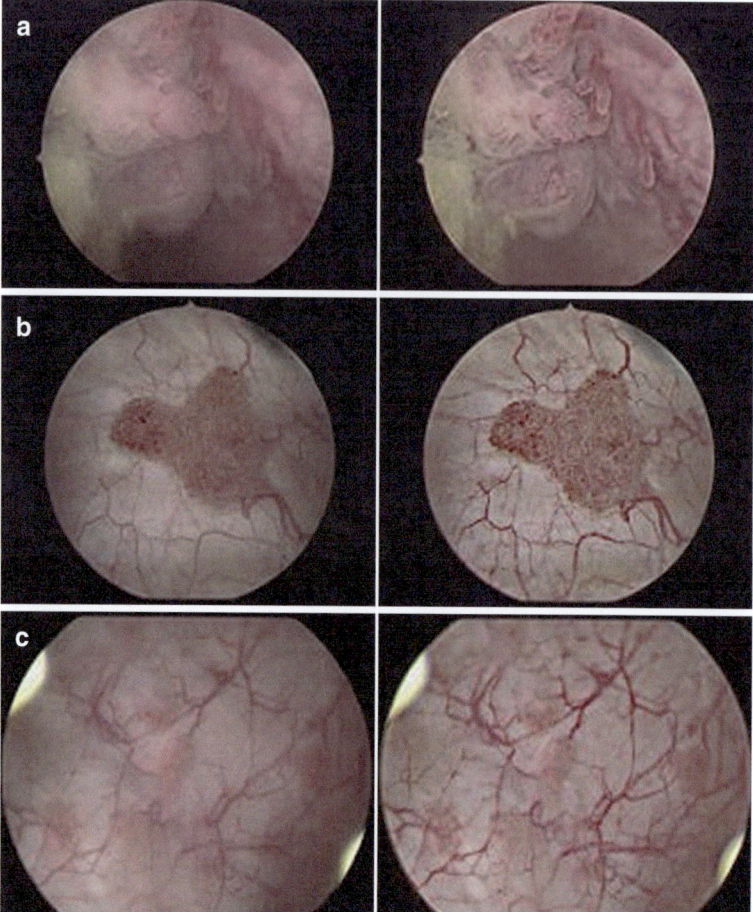

Fig. 11.10 Comparison of endoscopic visualization of various small polyps of the left renal pelvis in white light (*left*) and (**a**) Spectra A mode (*right*), (**b**) Spectra B mode (*right*) and (**c**) combined Chroma-Clara mode (*right*) (By courtesy of Dr. G Kamphuis and JJ de la Rosette)

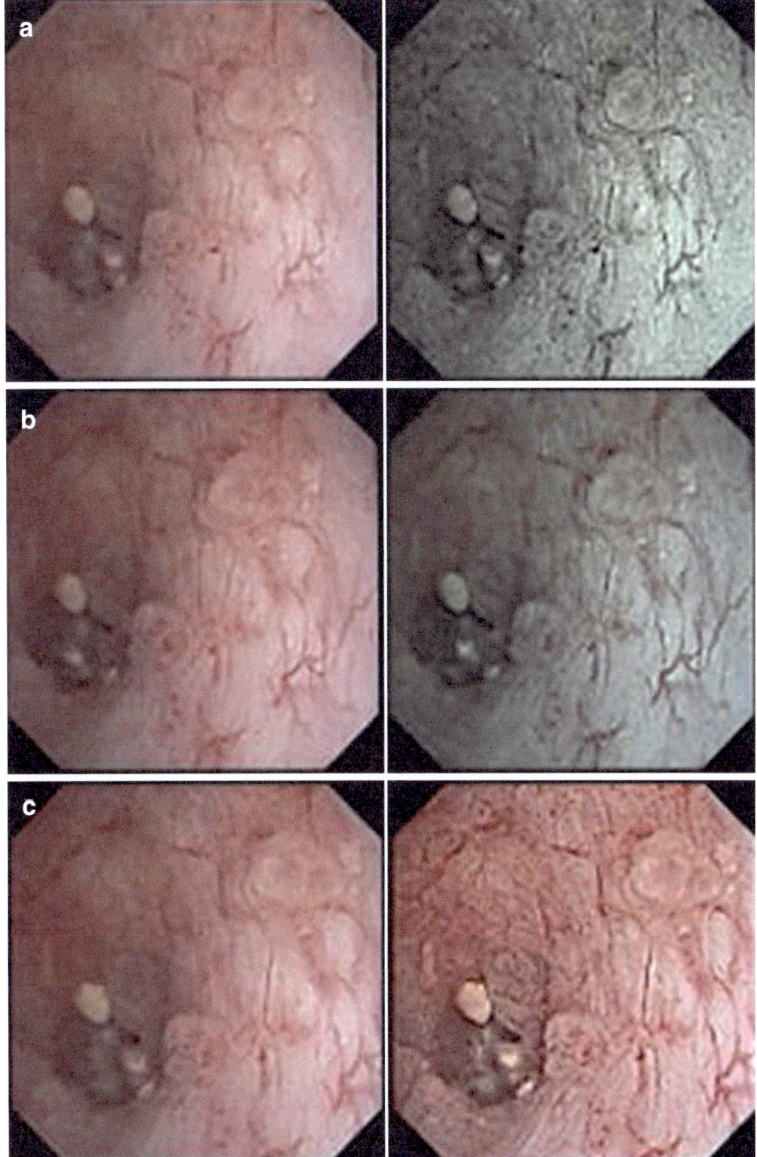

References

1. Humphreys MR, Miller NL, Williams Jr JC, Evan AP, Munch LC, Lingeman JE. A new world revealed: early experience with digital ureteroscopy. J Urol. 2008;179(3):970–5.
2. Andonian S, Okeke Z, Smith AD. Digital ureteroscopy: the next step. J Endourol. 2008;22(4):603–6. doi:10.1089/end.2008.0017.
3. Keeley FX, Kulp DA, Bibbo M, McCue PA, Bagley DH. Diagnostic accuracy of ureteroscopic biopsy in upper tract transitional cell carcinoma. J Urol. 1997; 157(1):33–7.
4. Smith AK, Stephenson AJ, Lane BR, et al. Inadequacy of biopsy for diagnosis of upper tract urothelial carcinoma: implications for conservative management. Urology. 2011;78(1):82–6.
5. Babjuk M, Burger M, Zigeuner R, et al. EAU guidelines on non-muscle-invasive urothelial carcinoma of the bladder: update 2013. Eur Urol. 2013;64(4): 639–53.
6. Gono K, Obi T, Yamaguchi M, Ohyama N, Machida H, Sano Y, Yoshida S, Hamamoto Y, Endo T. Appearance of enhanced tissue features in narrow-band endoscopic imaging. J Biomed Opt. 2004;9(3): 568–77.
7. Cauberg EC, Kloen S, Visser M, et al. Narrow band imaging cystoscopy improves the detection of non-muscle-invasive bladder cancer. Urology. 2010;76(3): 658–63.
8. Herr HW, Donat MS. A comparison of white-light cystoscopy and narrow-band imaging cystoscopy to detect bladder tumour recurrences. BJU Int. 2008;102:1111–14.
9. Bryan RT, Billingham LL, Wallace MA. Narrow-band imaging flexible cystoscopy in the detection of recurrent urothelial cancer of the bladder. BJU Int. 2008;101(6):702–5.
10. Naselli A, Introini C, Timossi L, Spina B, Fontana V, Pezzi R, Germinale F, Bertolotto F, Puppo P. A randomized prospective trial to assess the impact of transurethral resection in narrow band imaging modality on non-muscle-invasive bladder cancer recurrence. Eur Urol. 2012;61(5):908–13.
11. Traxer O, Geavlete B, de Medina SG, Sibony M, Al-Qahtani SM. Narrow-band imaging digital flexible ureteroscopy in detection of upper urinary tract transitional-cell carcinoma: initial experience. J Endourol. 2011;25(1):19–23.
12. Jocham D, Stepp H, Waidelich R. Photodynamic diagnosis in urology: state-of-the-art. Eur Urol. 2008;53:1138–48.
13. Batlle AM. Porphyrins, porphyrias, cancer and photodynamic therapy—a model for carcinogenesis. J Photochem Photobiol B. 1993;20:5–22.
14. Kennedy JC, Pottier RH. Endogenous protoporphyrin IX, a clinical useful photosensitizer for photodynamic therapy. J Photochem Photobiol B. 1992;14:275–92.
15. Kausch I, Sommerauer M, Montorsi F, et al. Photodynamic diagnosis in non-muscle-invasive bladder cancer: a systematic review and cumulative analysis of prospective studies. Eur Urol. 2010;57(4): 595–606.
16. Mowatt G, N'Dow J, Vale L, et al; Aberdeen Technology Assessment Review (TAR) Group. Photodynamic diagnosis of bladder cancer compared with white light cystoscopy: Systematic review and meta-analysis. Int J Technol Assess Health Care. 2011;27(1):3–10.
17. Omar M, Aboumarzouk OM, Mains E, Moseley H, Kata SG. Diagnosis of upper urinary tract tumours: is photodynamic diagnosis assisted ureterorenoscopy required as an addition to modern imaging and ureterorenoscopy? Photodiagnosis Photodyn Ther. 2013;10:127–33.
18. Marti A, Jichlinski P, Lange N, et al. Comparison of aminolevulinic acid and hexylester aminolevulinate induced protoporphyrin IX distribution in human bladder cancer. J Urol. 2003;170:428–32.
19. Frimberger D, Zaak D, Stepp H, et al. Autofluorescence imaging to optimize 5-ALA-induced fluorescence endoscopy of bladder carcinoma. Urology. 2001;58: 372–5.
20. Schäfauer C, Ettori D, Rouprêt M, et al. Detection of bladder urothelial carcinoma using in vivo noncontact, ultraviolet excited autofluorescence measurements converted into simple color coded images: a feasibility study. J Urol. 2013;190(1):271–7.

Beyond Endoscopy-Ultrasound, Optical Coherence Tomography and Confocal Laser Endomicroscopy

12

Mieke T.J. Bus, Daniel Martin de Bruin, Guido M. Kamphuis, Theo M. de Reijke, and Jean J.M.C.H. de la Rosette

12.1 Introduction

One of the main challenges in endoscopic diagnosis and treatment of upper urinary tract urothelial carcinoma is the complicated anatomy and the small size of the upper urinary tract, resulting in high demands on the armamentarium and expertise of the urologist. Difficulties to reach the complete collecting system could result in an incomplete visual inspection.

To reach the renal pelvis, the instruments have to pass the urethra (and prostate) and are then inserted through the ureteral orifice into the ureter. The ureter is a tubular structure that is generally 22–30 cm in length, 2–4 mm in width and

M.T.J. Bus, MD (✉) • G.M. Kamphuis, MD
T.M. de Reijke, MD, PhD
Jean J.M.C.H. de la Rosette, MD, PhD
Department of Urology, Academic Medical Center,
University of Amsterdam, Meibergdreef 9,
Amsterdam 1105 AZ, The Netherlands
e-mail: m.t.bus@amc.uva.nl;
g.m.kamphuis@amc.uva.nl;
t.m.dereyke@amc.uva.nl; j.j.delarosette@amc.uva.nl

D.M. de Bruin, PhD
Department of Urology, Academic Medical Center,
University of Amsterdam, Meibergdreef 9,
Amsterdam 1105 AZ, The Netherlands

Department of Biomedical Engineering and Physics,
Academic Medical Center, University of Amsterdam,
Meibergdreef 9, Amsterdam 1105 AZ,
The Netherlands
e-mail: d.m.debruin@amc.uva.nl

has a wall thickness of 350–750 μm. Anatomical angulation of the ureter may restrict the insertion of (semi-rigid and flexible) endoscopes, but also anatomical tapering of the ureter may provide difficulties. While inserting a ureterorenoscope in the ureter, one will come across three anatomical restrictions of the ureter. The first is the ureterovesical junction. The intramural ureter is compressed as it runs through the bladder wall and narrows considerably. The second region is located at the crossing of the ureter with the iliac vessels, caused by extrinsic compression of the iliac vessels. Finally, at the ureteropelvic junction, the proximal ureter is narrowed where it passes into the renal pelvis.

By using a flexible ureterorenoscope the renal pelvis and the major calyces can usually easily be reached. There is a huge anatomical variation in the number and location of the calyces and sometimes the necks of the calyces can also be narrow and not allowing the endoscope to enter. Therefore, visual inspection should always be combined with fluoroscopic imaging. To reach the lower pole calyx, the tip of the endoscope has to be capable to make a curve up to 180°. The major calyceal branches are formed by the infundibula. Each infundibulum runs to a minor calyx that divides into one or more individual papillae.

As depicted in Fig. 12.1, the anatomy of the upper urinary tract demands great flexibility of the endoscopes and instruments to inspect and treat the complete collecting system. The limited

© Springer International Publishing Switzerland 2015
M. Grasso III, D.H. Bagley (eds.), *Upper Urinary Tract Urothelial Carcinoma*,
DOI 10.1007/978-3-319-13869-5_12

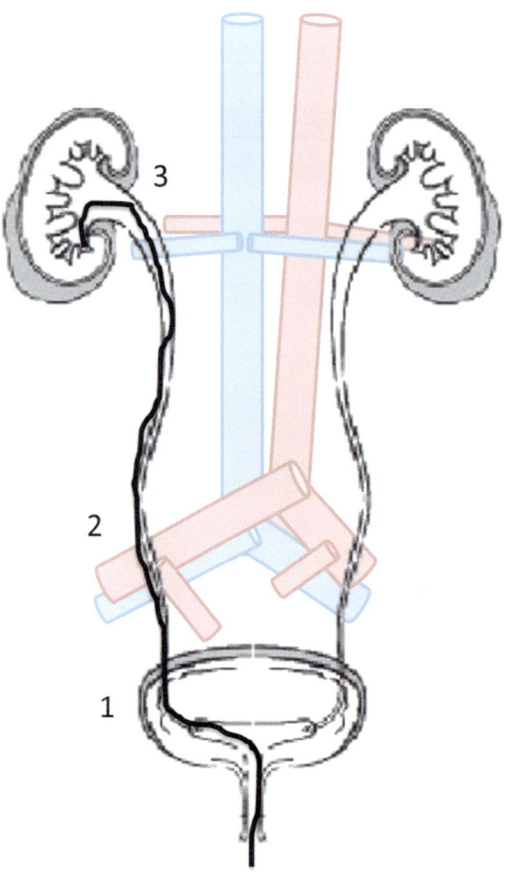

Fig. 12.1 Anatomy of the upper urinary tract demonstrating the anatomical restrictions in the upper urinary tract. The intramural ureter is compressed as it runs through the bladder wall and narrows considerably at the ureterovesical junction (*1*). By extrinsic compression of the iliac vessels, the crossing ureter is narrowed (*2*) and at the ureteropelvic junction (*3*) the proximal ureter is narrowed where it passes into the renal pelvis

diameter of the ureter, however, considerably limits the size of the instruments that can be used in the upper urinary tract through the (flexible) ureterorenoscopes. Semi-rigid ureterorenoscopes are available in a wide variety and diameters ranging from 4.5 to 11.5 Fr. There are models that consist of a one sized diameter and models that increase in diameter from tip to proximal. Semi-rigid scopes can be used to visualize the distal, middle and proximal ureter. However, to visualize the complete upper urinary tract including pyelum, calyxes and papillae, flexible ureterorenoscopy should be performed in combination

with semi-rigid endoscopy. Modern flexible ureterorenoscopes have a tip diameter of 4.9–8.7 Fr, a shaft diameter of 7.1–10.9 Fr and a proximal diameter of 7.2–10.9 Fr. Modern flexible ureterorenoscopes can reach a deflection of up to 275° [1]. Besides diameter of the scope, the diameter of the working channel is of importance, as it is used for irrigation with water as well as for placement of instruments like graspers, baskets and laser fibers. Introducing these instruments reduces the irrigation considerably and therefore dedicated irrigation aids are being used, necessary for optimal viewing.

In case of a suspect lesion, histopathological examination is mandatory. Biopsy specimens retrieved during ureterorenoscopy are frequently minute because of the application of small caliber instruments [2], and may therefore be difficult to examine by the pathologist. Consequently, a high rate of tumour upgrading (37–96 %) and upstaging (38 %) is reported following nephroureterectomy [3, 4]. Over the past decade, conservative endoscopic treatment has gained increased interest for a selected group of patients with upper urinary tract urothelial carcinoma (UUT-UC), not only in case of a mandatory indication (patients with a solitary kidney), but also for patients with low-volume, low-grade, low stage disease [5, 6] and a healthy contralateral kidney. Although radical nephroureterectomy (including bladder cuff) is the gold standard in the treatment of UUT-UC, estimated Glomerular Filtration Rate (eGFR) decreases significantly in patients with UUT-UC after nephroureterectomy [7–9] and chronic kidney disease (CKD) is associated with a significant increase in cardiovascular events and death of any cause, independent of co-existing comorbidities [10]. For this reason endoscopic treatment is more accepted in patients with low-risk disease.

To decide which patients are eligible for endoscopic treatment, information on tumour stage and grade has become imminent for clinical decision-making. Optimizing endoscopic visualization and accurate diagnosis of UUT-UC is therefore a prerequisite. Novel optical diagnostic techniques, based on the interaction of light with tissue, have the potential to improve this visualization and diagnosis of UUT-UC [11]. These interactions include scattering, absorption and fluorescence, all of which are characteristic for certain tissue types. Some of these techniques aim to provide real time intra-operative information on tumour grade and stage. If knowledge about tumour grade and stage is obtained during URS, a better selection of patients eligible for endoscopic treatment is possible and safe and simultaneous treatment can be applied. It is because of this promise that optical diagnostics might reduce the limitations of the current biopsies.

Most research on the application of optical diagnostics on urothelium has been done in the field of bladder cancer [12, 13]. Results on bladder urothelium resemble ureteral urothelium. However, the limited space in the ureter and the difficulty of reaching the upper urinary tract creates a whole new spectrum of challenges for the applied optical techniques. Given the speed of current technical developments and miniaturization, optical diagnostics have become available for the diagnostic work up of upper urinary tract investigation.

12.2 Endoluminal Ultrasound (ELUS)

Endoluminal Ultrasound (ELUS) is an imaging technique that can be applied in a variety of luminal structures. ELUS is based on detecting an echo time delay of high frequency sound waves, which are backscattered by structures in tissue. Plotting of the reflecting ultrasound amplitude vs depth composes endoluminal images. The most common examples of endoluminal ultrasound are intravascular ultrasound, transvaginal ultrasound and transrectal ultrasound. Advances of this technique has led to small catheter-based ultrasound probes allowing visualization of a variety of other luminal structures, such as bile ducts, fallopian tubes, small bowel, oesophagus and blood vessels [14, 15]. Current ultrasound probes consist of flexible 2.4 mm diameter (7.2 F) catheters

containing a 12.5 or 20 MHz transducer (Olympus, Tokyo, Japan) [16]. ELUS probes designed for use in the upper urinary tract have a hole through the end for placement over a Terumo guide-wire. The ultrasound probes are re-usable and can be sterilized in the same way as standard endoscopy equipment. The ultrasound transducer is attached to a motor that continually rotates providing real-time 360° cross-sectional images of the ureteric wall and surrounding structures and a pullback allowing 3D imaging of a UUT segment. Imaging penetration depth is dependent on the frequency of the ultrasound transducer. The 12.5 MHz transducer enables axial imaging with a penetration depth of maximum 40 mm around the ureter. The 20 MHz transducer enables axial imaging with a penetration depth of maximal 20 mm from the centre of the transducer and provides an axial resolution of 100 μm (Olympus, Tokyo, Japan) [16].

The transmission of sound waves needs a conducting medium. This restricts imaging to fluid filled structures, such as the lumen of the upper urinary tract. However, air bubbles introduced accidentally in the irrigation water due to the procedure create large back scattering, disturbing signals. An advantage of endoluminal ultrasound is its deeper imaging depth compared to other endoluminal imaging techniques (Table 12.1) which can be helpful to determine the relation of specific pathologies with its direct surroundings, like increased lymph nodes in malignancies [16]. In the ureter, endoluminal ultrasound has mainly been used for the treatment of UPJ stenosis, when an endoluminal incision was considered and the location of crossing vessels had to be determined. By using ELUS, the exact location of crossing vessels can be determined and therefore the best incision plane can be chosen [17]. Other possible indications for ELUS are identification and staging of upper urinary tract tumours, submucosal calculi, endometriosis and inflammation [16, 18] (Fig. 12.2).

However, improvement of CT imaging has led to a decrease of the use of ELUS in the field of urology, because it is less invasive and considerable costs are involved.

Table 12.1 Overview of the three endoluminal diagnostic techniques, including imaging depth and resolution

	Principle	Purposes	Imaging depth	Resolution (μm)	Advantage	Limitations
ELUS	Sound scattering	Real time imaging of luminal structures	20–40 mm	100	High imaging penetration depth	Low resolution images movement artefacts low data aquisition speed
OCT	Light scatteringc	Real time information on pathohistological diagnosis	2–3 mm	20	Information on tumour grade and stage suitable for screening purposus of complete ureter fast data aquisition speed	Diminished imaging depth range
CLE	Absorption/ reflection	Real time information on pathohistological diagnosis	400 μm	3.5	In-vivo microscopy with high resolution images	Sensitivity to tissue movement additional staining needed

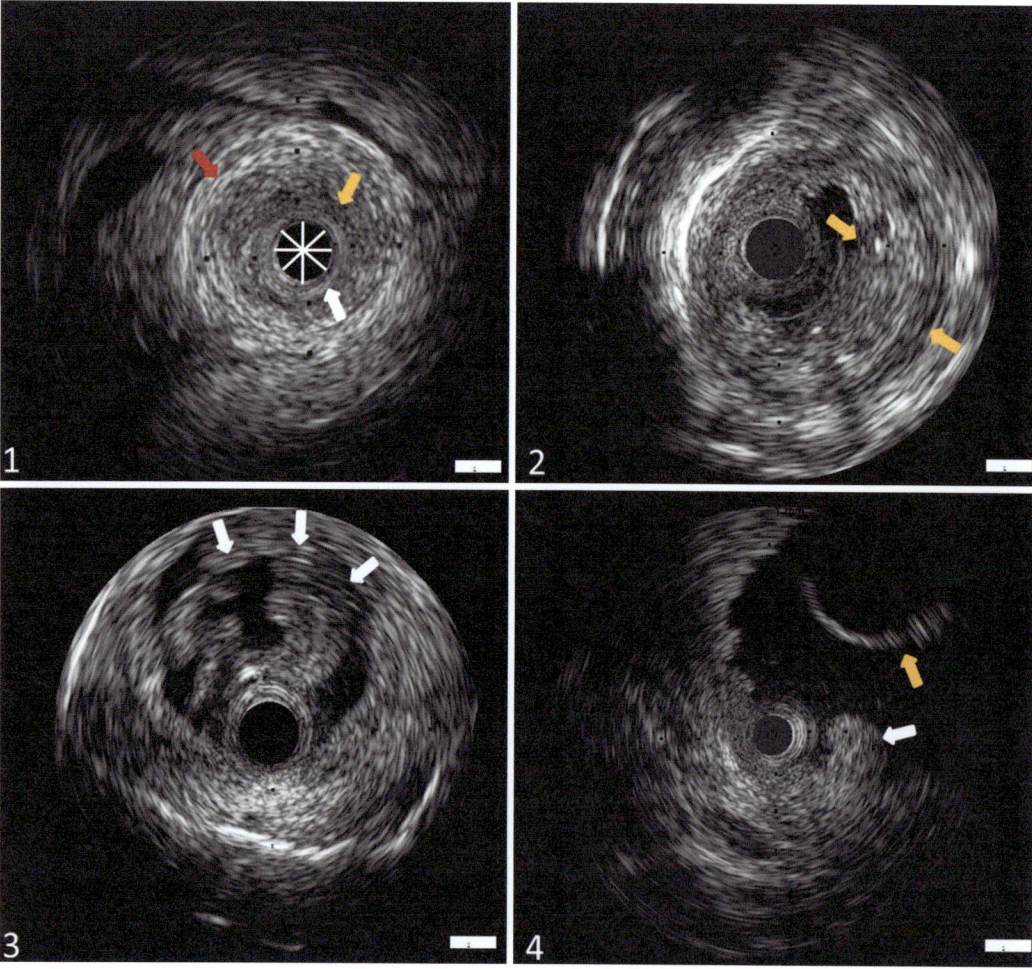

Fig. 12.2 Ex-vivo cross-sectional images of the ureter and pyelum using endoluminal ultrasound (ELUS). (*1*) ELUS image of normal appearing ureter, demonstrating inner hyperechoic mucosa (*white arrow*), hypoechoic muscularis (*orange arrow*) and hyperechoic periureteric fat (*red arrow*). The probe is indicated in this figure (⁕). (*2*) ELUS image of the ureter demonstrating solid urothelial carcinoma (T1G3) showing irregular thickened mucosal layer. (*3*) ELUS image of a TaG1 papillary urothelial carcinoma of the ureter (*white arrows*). (*4*) ELUS image of the pyelum, showing an invasive high-grade urothelial carcinoma (*white arrow*) and nephrostomy tube (*orange arrow*)

12.3   Optical Coherence Tomography

Optical Coherence Tomography (OCT) is a high resolution imaging technology originally applied in ophthalmology [19]. OCT is analogous to ultrasonography, using back-scattered light instead of back-scattered sound waves to produce micrometer-scale resolution, cross-sectional images (Fig. 12.3). "State of the art" OCT research investigates the position of this relative novel technology in the diagnostic workup of several epithelial cancers [20, 21]. The use of optical fibers allows OCT to be applied endoluminally through the working channel of small calibre rigid and flexible endoscopes. The commercially available OCT imaging probe currently

at use for upper urinary tract imaging is originally designed for cardiovascular applications. For this reason, the 0.9 mm (2.7 Fr) fiber has to be interfaced with an intravascular imaging system. This automatic pullback system scans a longitudinal trajectory of 54 mm in approximately 5.4 s, producing a 540-frame dataset at 20 μm axial resolution. In OCT images of the urinary bladder wall, layered tissue anatomy can be distinguished, e.g., the basement membrane, which integrity is indicative of low stage in case a bladder tumour is identified [22]. Additionally, the light scattering causes a decrease of OCT signal magnitude over depth, and limits the imaging range to approximately 2 mm depth. This rate of OCT signal decrease with depth is quantified by the attenuation coefficient (μ_{oct}) that allows

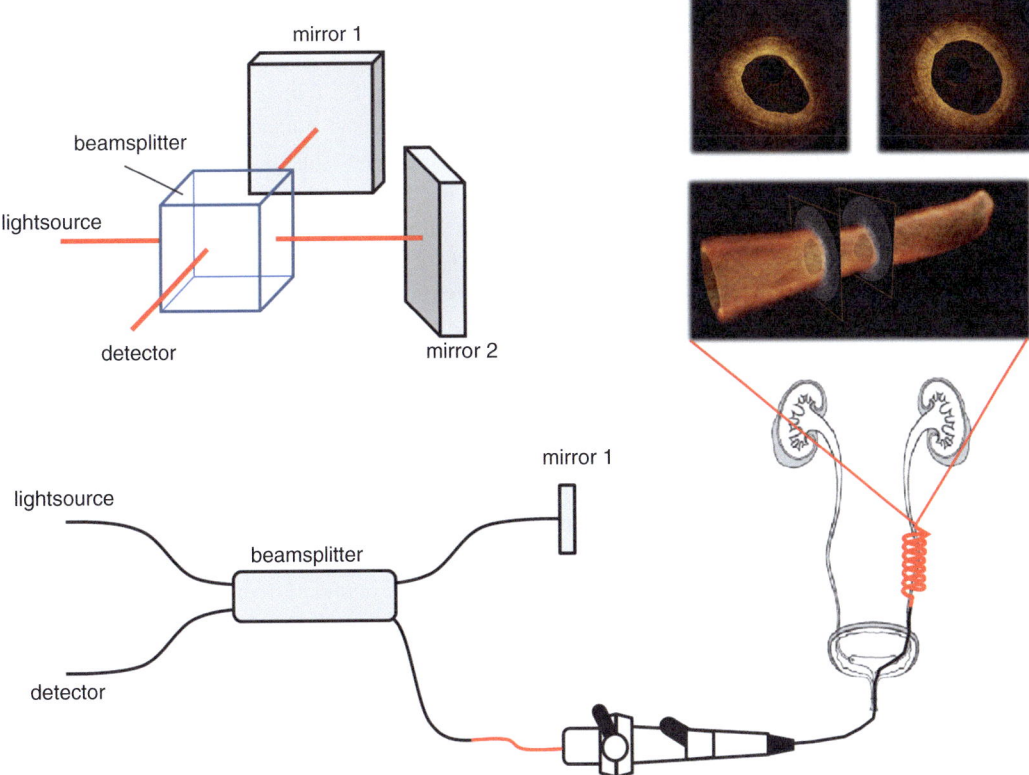

Fig. 12.3 Optical Coherence Tomography (OCT) is the optical equivalent of ultrasound imaging, measuring light reflectivity vs. depth. It is based on white light (large wavelength bandwidth) interferometry, where interference signals are only detected if the light in the sample and reference arm has travelled equal distances. Thus, by varying the length of the reference arm, the imaging location in the tissue can be controlled. Modern embodiments of OCT do not use moving reference mirrors; instead technical complexity is shifted towards either the light source (that sequentially provides each wavelength within the source bandwidth at high speed) or the detector (which detects each wavelength within the source bandwidth in parallel)

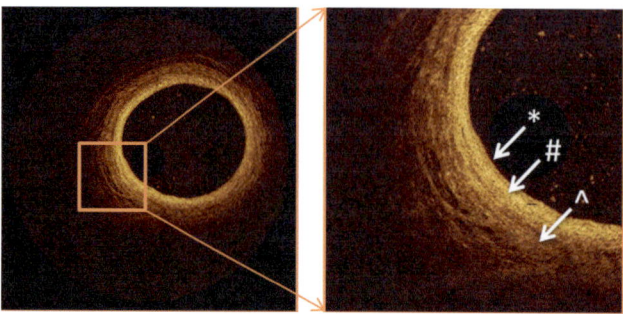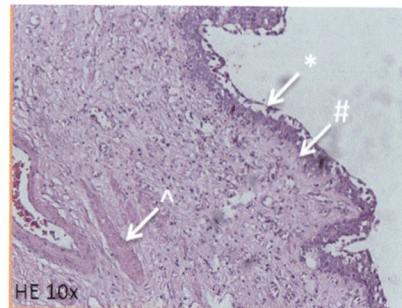

Fig. 12.4 Optical Coherence Tomography image of a normal ureter, showing anatomical layers of the ureter wall compared to histological image of the normal ureter. The layers of the ureter can clearly be recognized. * urothelium, # lamina propria, ^ muscularis propria

in-vivo differentiation between different tissue types [21, 23–25]. This distinction results from differences in intra- and extracellular organization of the tissue, which is reflected in the light scattering properties. Measurement of μ_{oct} could therefore discriminate differences in organization that could be associated with different grades of the lesion. This has theoretically been described and tested in an animal study by Xie et al. [26], where they showed differences in scattering properties between normal and malignant bladder urothelium.

The potential of OCT for staging and diagnosis of UUT-UC has been investigated ex-vivo in the porcine ureter and these investigations demonstrated that OCT can clearly distinguish the ureteral wall layers, particularly the urothelium and lamina propria [27, 28]. When compared to endoluminal ultrasonography, OCT significantly better distinguishes the wall layers of ex-vivo porcine ureter [29]. An in-vivo human pilot study showed that normal appearing urothelium including basal membrane, CIS and visible protrusions could be visualized on OCT images (Fig. 12.4). Additionally, OCT is able to visually differentiate between non-invasive and invasive tumours (Fig. 12.5) and it can differentiate between low- and high-grade lesions by quantifying μ_{oct} [30]. However, current OCT analyses cannot obtain a reliable μ_{oct} from normal appearing urothelium or CIS due to the limited thickness of these layers (around 50 μm). Improvement by increasing the resolution of OCT could solve this limitation. Recently published novel attenuation analysis

methods for thin layers could solve this limitation, but these methods do require additional research since it is still in an early stage of development [31].

Several features of OCT are appealing for intraluminal diagnostics. First, flexible OCT probes are compatible with modern endoscopes and easy to apply in the ureter, pyelum and calyces, enabling OCT imaging at all sites within the urinary tract and not interfering with deflecting properties and rinsing during the procedure. Second, OCT measurement duration per patient adds only maximal five minutes operating time during URS, as the probe is easy to use and a single measurement takes 5.4 s per region under investigation. Third, OCT does not require a conducting medium or direct contact, which makes it easily applicable in the ureter. Finally, the OCT system is compact and portable, which results in an easy to use system in the operating theatre. In conclusion, the advantages of OCT are the non-invasive, real-time and high-resolution 3D imaging that allows visual staging and extraction of the optical attenuation coefficient that allows grading. However, current commercial available OCT systems are limited to image a lumen with a maximal diameter of 10 mm, compromising visualization of the pyelum and bladder as a whole. Furthermore, if tumour thickness transcends scattering-limited imaging depth in tissue (~2 mm), invasiveness cannot be assessed. A recent study quantified the learning curve and inter-observer variance of the μ_{oct}. It was concluded that routine μ_{oct} determination for tissue

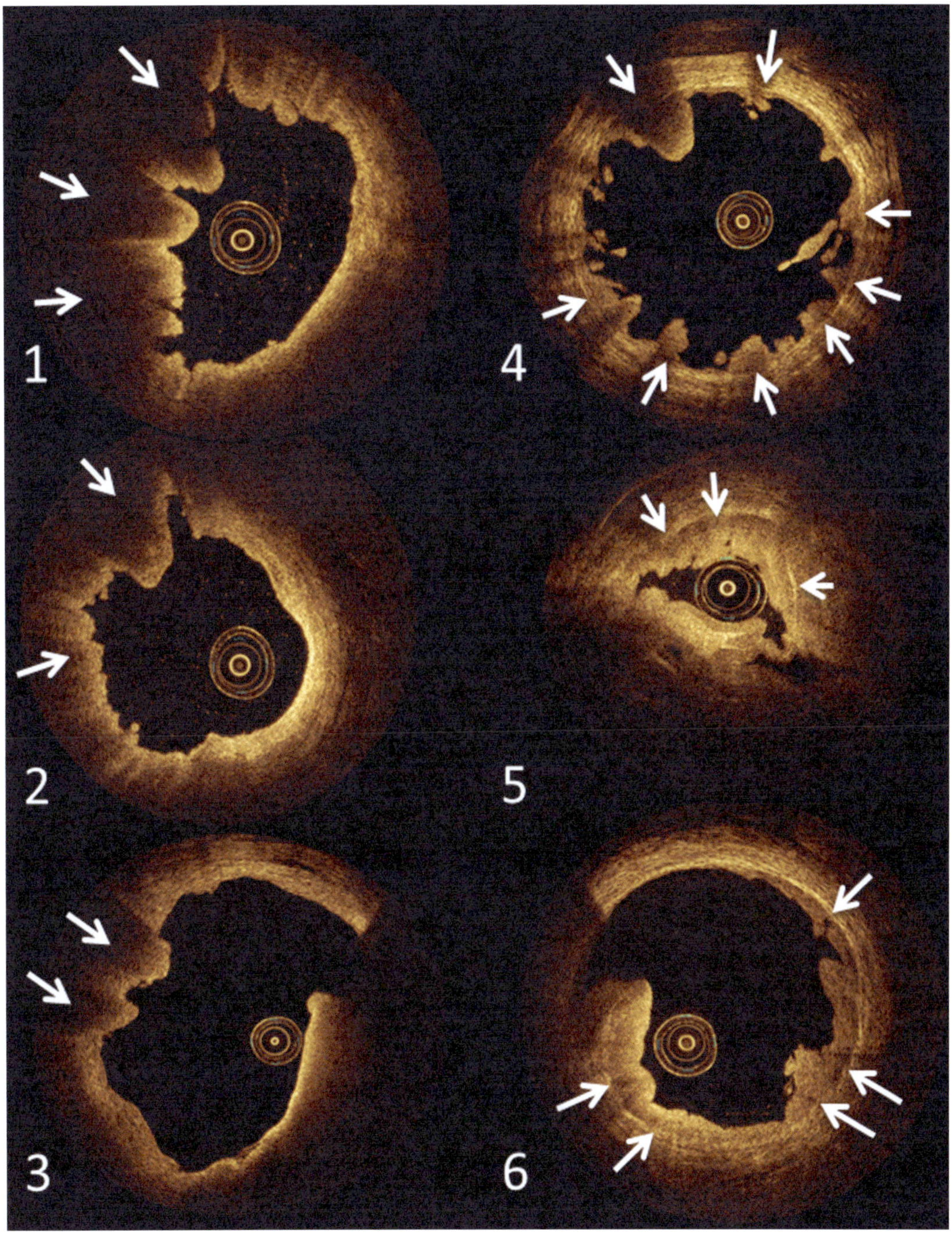

Fig. 12.5 Upper urinary tract urothelial carcinoma as seen with optical coherence tomography imaging. (*1–3*) Represent invasive UUT-UC. Invasive UUT-UC (≥T1) can be recognized as a loss of architecture of the anatomical layers underneath visible layers. (*4–6*) Demonstrate non-invasive UUT-UC. Underneath the visible tumour lesions the anatomical layering of the ureter wall can be clearly recognized

classification does not require extensive training and that OCT naïve people only require three trainings to acquire the same results as experienced OCT investigators. This increases the clinical potential of OCT [32].

12.4   Confocal Laser Endomicroscopy

Confocal Laser Endomicroscopy (CLE) is an optical technique originally applied in cell-biology. CLE allows for ultra-high resolution microscopy of tissue up to an imaging depth of 400 µm. This imaging depth and resolution can be achieved using lasers and optics which are combined with a very small hole (pin-hole) that acts as a diaphragm in the microscope objective (Fig. 12.6). This special microscope lens ensures that only light from the focus in the tissue is collected. All the other light that is out of focus is rejected by the pinhole. The imaging depth of CLE is therefore much higher than normal microscopy that is typically limited to 20 µm because of out-of-focus blurring (i.e., the thickness of a histology slide). While conventional confocal microscopes are too large to use in vivo, recent advantages in instrument miniaturization have led to the development of flexible, fiberoptic confocal microscopes that can be used with standard endoscopy. This creates confocal endomicroscopes that can be used in environments such as the bladder to study the cellular structure of the bladder wall. Combining confocal microscopy with fluorescent probes creates additional contrast. The fluorescent probe emits light that is filtered through the pinhole so that only in-focus light is measured by the photodetector while the out of focus light is rejected. This results in optimal sectioning of the regions of interest with micron-scale resolution, which allows cellular differentiation [33]. The tissue can be stained non-specifically, commonly using fluorescein as fluorescent probe. This FDA approved contrast agent can be administered intravenously or topically and rapidly stains the extracellular matrix. CLE has been studied in vivo in the urinary bladder. Endomicroscopy images visualized excellent the umbrella cells, intermediate cells, lamina propria including blood vessels filled with erythrocytes. Fibers of the muscularis propria and perivesical fat images could be obtained from the tumour resection bed. Secondly, the images demonstrated clear differences between normal urothelium, low-, and high-grade tumours [34, 35]. However, a major drawback of this technique is the sensitivity to tissue movement due to the long acquisition time, resulting in blurred images.

High resolution of 1 µm and a field of view of 240 µm have been achieved with probes with a diameter of 2.6 mm (7.8 Fr), which can only be inserted through a rigid cystoscope. Since the probe requires direct contact with the tissue, some tumours located at the anterior and lateral bladder wall cannot be visualized with CLE [34]. A study with a 1.4 mm (4.2 Fr) diameter probe, which can be inserted through the working channel of a flexible cystoscope, overcomes this hurdle. Both probes are capable of providing histological images. The 1.4 mm probe has a wider field of view (600 µm) and results in improved imaging of the microarchitecture compared to the 2.6 mm probe. However, since the resolution of this 1.4 mm probe is 3.5 µm, the cellular resolution essential for diagnosis that the 2.6 mm probe provided could not be obtained with the 1.4 mm probe [36]. For implementation of CLE in the upper urinary tract, smaller imaging probes compatible with flexible ureterorenoscopes are needed to obtain direct contact of the probe with tissue and optimal resolution. An ex-vivo study in the renal pelvis and proximal ureter of nephrectomy specimens showed similar results as obtained from bladder images. Urothelial cells and lamina propria were clearly recognized [35]. Recently a 0.85 mm (2.55 Fr) imaging probe compatible with semi-rigid and flexible ureterorenoscopes became available, allowing CLE imaging in the upper urinary tract. Like the 1.4 mm imaging probe, this probe demonstrates a lower resolution of 3.5 µm compared to the 2.6 mm imaging probe. A high resolution is needed identifying all the diagnostic features. However, an initial study on CLE in the upper urinary tract using this 0.85 mm imaging probe could image normal urothelium (Fig. 12.7, 1). In addition, imaging of UUT-UC showed characteristic features of tumours, including pleomorphic cells, fibro vascular stalks and papillary structures, despite the lower resolution (Fig. 12.7, 2) [33].

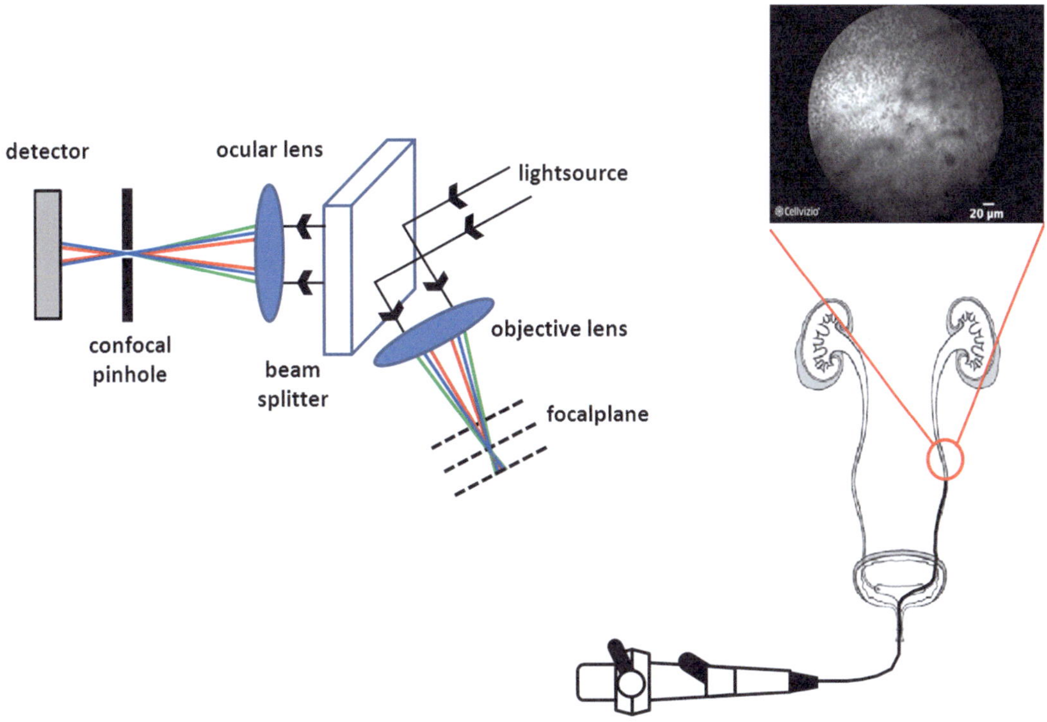

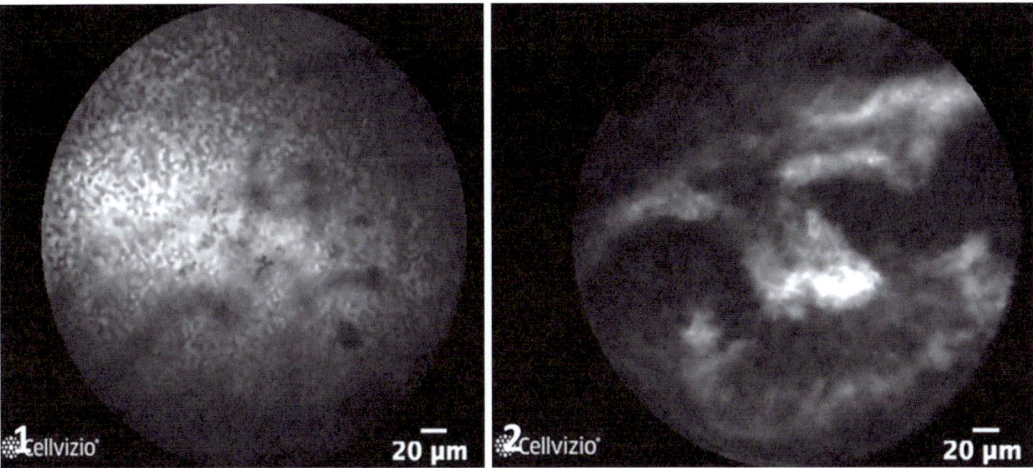

Fig. 12.6 Confocal Laser Endomicroscopy (CLE) is based on the suppression of out-of-focus light by the insertion of a pin-hole before the detector. This results in the detection of backscattered light that originates from the focal plane only (*red* and *blue* in the overview) while light that is backscattered outside the focal plane (*green* in the overview) is stopped by the pin-hole. Miniaturization of a confocal microscope affects the numerical aperture of the system, which will directly influence the resolution of the system. Insert shows ex-vivo CLE of normal proximal ureter from a radical nephrectomy specimen. Normal urothelium showing uniform, monomorphic cells consistent with intermediate cells

Fig. 12.7 Ureter wall imaged using confocal laser endomicroscopy (CLE). (*1*) Depicts normal urothelium as seen on CLE images. (*2*) Depicts low-grade upper urinary tract carcinoma as seen on CLE image (Images courtesy of Prof. O. Traxer, Université Pierre et Marie Curie, Tenon Hospital, Paris)

12.5 Future Perspectives on Technology Integration

Endoscopy in the upper urinary tract is challenging due to its small diameter and vulnerability of tissues. This environment creates many limitations that have to be tackled before endoluminal diagnostics can be reliably applied in the upper urinary tract. Although promising, OCT and CLE are new endoluminal diagnostic techniques and the additional diagnostic value has not been determined yet. In addition, cost effectiveness has not been determined for these new diagnostic techniques. Since the probe that is used in OCT is single use and the CLE probe has a limited use of six to eight times, the latest endoluminal diagnostics are costly. However, it can be hypothesized that histological diagnosis of UUT-UC will diminish the total amount of procedures and total costs, but studies about the costs in UUT-UC management should confirm this hypothesis.

From a clinical point of view, the ideal adjunct modality for endoscopic procedures in the upper urinary tract should: (1) increase the sensitivity and specificity of detecting malignant and premalignant lesions, (2) provide reliable information on grade and stage, (3) reliably identify the lateral and deep margins in order to achieve complete resection and consequently identify residual tumour within resection margins, (4) easily integrate in modern ureterorenoscopes, (5) be easy to apply with a short learning curve for image interpretation, (6) not require the use of toxic or inconvenient chemicals or pharmaceuticals, (7) allow simultaneous display of a conventional white light image such that endoscopic surgery could be guided by such modality in real time, (8) be compact and easy to handle in the operation room and (9) preferably be low in additional costs [13, 36].

Although the combination of endoscopy and the diagnostic techniques described in this chapter show potential to improve diagnosis and therapy of UUT tumours, none of the described techniques in this overview meets all these conditions (Table 12.1). A disadvantage of ELUS is the time needed for data acquisition, which is a factor 20 longer, compared to data acquisition using OCT. This increased acquisition time makes ELUS more sensitive for movements, which results in blurred images. In an in-vivo setting movements will occur due to ureteric peristalsis, breathing and movement at the point where the ureter crosses the iliac vessels. In addition, ELUS has a lower resolution compared to the high-resolution of CLE and OCT. Although CLE and OCT produce high-resolution histology like images, they are limited in imaging depth. This hampers visualizing the pyelum as a whole. In addition, if tumour thickness transcends the imaging depth of these techniques, tumour invasiveness cannot be reliably assessed.

Furthermore, OCT, ELUS and CLE do not increase tumour detection rates. In the absence of visually suspect lesions, these techniques have to be used in combination with other methods to direct the imaging probes to regions of interest. A combination of image enhancement techniques, including narrow band imaging (NBI), photodynamic diagnosis (PDD), and SPIES could be such a real-time optical adjunct modality.

NBI is an optical image enhancement technique designed for endoscopic applications, with demonstrated value in gastroenterology and urology [37, 38]. NBI takes advantage of altered blood vessel morphology of mucosa to enhance contrast between mucosa and microvascular structures. This technique is based on the principle that the depth of light penetration into the mucosa increases with increasing wavelength. By illuminating the tissue surface with specific wavelengths (blue 415 nm and green 540 nm), both strongly absorbed by haemoglobin, the vascular structures appear dark brown/green against a pink/white mucosal background. This contrast enhancement can therefore result in improved tumour detection rates compared to white light endoscopy [39]. In the combination of NBI with for example OCT, NBI could be used first to visualize or target a suspected lesion and OCT could assist in epithelial lesion differentiation by addressing grade and stage as shown by several studies [21, 23, 30]. Similar considerations apply for the combination of NBI with CLE.

In conclusion, technical improvements have been introduced in the design of ureterorenoscopy armamentarium over the past 10 years. Modern (flexible) ureterorenoscopy results in improved visualization of upper urinary tract urothelial carcinoma. This has paved the way to allow endoscopic treatment of UUT-UC, starting in imperative indications and now expanding to elective indications. To overcome the problem of undergrading and understaging new optical diagnostics (optical coherence tomography and confocal laser endomicroscopy) are being evaluated in the upper urinary tract. In the future, a combination of optical diagnostics, optical enhancement techniques and improved ureterorenoscopy techniques should provide an optimal grading and staging of UUT-UC.

Acknowledgements The authors like to thank Prof. O. Traxer, Pierre et Marie Curie University, Tenon Hospital, France, for generously providing the confocal laser endomicroscopy images.

References

1. Al-Qahtani SM, Letendre J, Thomas A, Natalin R, Saussez T, Traxer O. Which ureteral access sheath is compatible with your flexible ureteroscope? J Endourol. 2014;28:286–90.
2. Tavora F, Fajardo DA, Lee TK, et al. Small endoscopic biopsies of the ureter and renal pelvis: pathologic pitfalls. Am J Surg Pathol. 2009;33:1540–6.
3. Wang JK, Tollefson MK, Krambeck AE, Trost LW, Thompson RH. High rate of pathologic upgrading at nephroureterectomy for upper tract urothelial carcinoma. Urology. 2012;79:615–9.
4. Smith AK, Stephenson AJ, Lane BR, et al. Inadequacy of biopsy for diagnosis of upper tract urothelial carcinoma: implications for conservative management. Urology. 2011;78:82–6.
5. Roupret M, Babjuk M, Comperat E, et al. European guidelines on upper tract urothelial carcinomas: 2013 update. Eur Urol. 2013;63:1059–71.
6. Ristau BT, Tomaszewski JJ, Ost MC. Upper tract urothelial carcinoma: current treatment and outcomes. Urology. 2012;79:749–56.
7. Lane BR, Smith AK, Larson BT, et al. Chronic kidney disease after nephroureterectomy for upper tract urothelial carcinoma and implications for the administration of perioperative chemotherapy. Cancer. 2010;116: 2967–73.
8. Xylinas E, Rink M, Margulis V, et al. Impact of renal function on eligibility for chemotherapy and survival in patients who have undergone radical nephroureterectomy. BJU Int. 2013;112:453–61.
9. Kaag MG, O'Malley RL, O'Malley P, et al. Changes in renal function following nephroureterectomy may affect the use of perioperative chemotherapy. Eur Urol. 2010;58:581–7.
10. Go AS, Chertow GM, Fan D, McCulloch CE, Hsu CY. Chronic kidney disease and the risks of death, cardiovascular events, and hospitalization. N Engl J Med. 2004;351:1296–305.
11. Bus MT, de Bruin DM, Faber DJ, et al. Optical diagnostics for upper urinary tract urothelial cancer: technology, thresholds and clinical applications. J Endourol. 2015;29:113–23.
12. Cauberg EC, de Bruin DM, Faber DJ, van Leeuwen TG, de la Rosette JJ, de Reijke TM. A new generation of optical diagnostics for bladder cancer: technology, diagnostic accuracy, and future applications. Eur Urol. 2009;56:287–96.
13. Liu JJ, Droller MJ, Liao JC. New optical imaging technologies for bladder cancer: considerations and perspectives. J Urol. 2012;188:361–8.
14. Goldberg BB, Liu JB, Merton DA, Kurtz AB. Endoluminal US: experiments with nonvascular uses in animals. Radiology. 1990;175:39–43.
15. Hodgson JM, Graham SP, Savakus AD, et al. Clinical percutaneous imaging of coronary anatomy using an over-the-wire ultrasound catheter system. Int J Card Imaging. 1989;4:187–93.
16. Ingram MD, Sooriakumaran P, Palfrey E, Montgomery B, Massouh H. Evaluation of the upper urinary tract using transureteric ultrasound–a review of the technique and typical imaging appearances. Clin Radiol. 2008;63:1026–34.
17. Hendrikx AJ, Nadorp S, De Beer NA, Van Beekum JB, Gravas S. The use of endoluminal ultrasonography for preventing significant bleeding during endopyelotomy: evaluation of helical computed tomography vs endoluminal ultrasonography for detecting crossing vessels. BJU Int. 2006;97:786–9.
18. Goldberg BB, Bagley D, Liu JB, Merton DA, Alexander A, Kurtz AB. Endoluminal sonography of the urinary tract: preliminary observations. AJR Am J Roentgenol. 1991;156:99–103.
19. Huang D, Swanson EA, Lin CP, et al. Optical coherence tomography. Science. 1991;254:1178–81.
20. Vakoc BJ, Lanning RM, Tyrrell JA, et al. Three-dimensional microscopy of the tumor microenvironment in vivo using optical frequency domain imaging. Nat Med. 2009;15:1219–23.
21. Wessels R, de Bruin DM, Faber DJ, et al. Optical coherence tomography in vulvar intraepithelial neoplasia. J Biomed Opt. 2012;17:116022.
22. Hermes B, Spoler F, Naami A, et al. Visualization of the basement membrane zone of the bladder by optical coherence tomography: feasibility of noninvasive evaluation of tumor invasion. Urology. 2008;72:677–81.
23. Barwari K, de Bruin DM, Faber DJ, van Leeuwen TG, de la Rosette JJ, Laguna MP. Differentiation between normal renal tissue and renal tumours using functional optical coherence tomography: a phase I in vivo human study. BJU Int. 2012;110:E415–20.

24. McLaughlin RA, Scolaro L, Robbins P, Saunders C, Jacques SL, Sampson DD. Mapping tissue optical attenuation to identify cancer using optical coherence tomography. Med Image Comput Comput Assist Interv. 2009;12:657–64.

25. Tomlins PH, Adegun O, Hagi-Pavli E, Piper K, Bader D, Fortune F. Scattering attenuation microscopy of oral epithelial dysplasia. J Biomed Opt. 2010;15:066003.

26. Xie T, Zeidel M, Pan Y. Detection of tumorigenesis in urinary bladder with optical coherence tomography: optical characterization of morphological changes. Opt Express. 2002;10:1431–43.

27. Mueller-Lisse UL, Meissner OA, Babaryka G, et al. Catheter-based intraluminal optical coherence tomography (OCT) of the ureter: ex-vivo correlation with histology in porcine specimens. Eur Radiol. 2006;16:2259–64.

28. Wang H, Kang W, Zhu H, MacLennan G, Rollins AM. Three-dimensional imaging of ureter with endoscopic optical coherence tomography. Urology. 2011;77:1254–8.

29. Mueller-Lisse UL, Meissner OA, Bauer M, et al. Catheter-based intraluminal optical coherence tomography versus endoluminal ultrasonography of porcine ureter ex vivo. Urology. 2009;73:1388–91.

30. Bus MT, Muller BG, de Bruin DM, et al. Volumetric in vivo visualization of upper urinary tract tumors using optical coherence tomography: a pilot study. J Urol. 2013;190:2236–42.

31. Vermeer KA, Mo J, Weda JJ, Lemij HG, de Boer JF. Depth-resolved model-based reconstruction of attenuation coefficients in optical coherence tomography. Biomed Opt Express. 2013;5:322–37.

32. Wessels R, de Bruin DM, Faber DJ, et al. Inter observer variance and learning curve in quantification of the optical coherence tomography attenuation coefficient. J Biomed Opt. 2015.

33. Chen SP, Liao JC. Confocal laser endomicroscopy of bladder and upper tract urothelial carcinoma: a new era of optical diagnosis? Curr Urol Rep. 2014; 15:437.

34. Sonn GA, Jones SN, Tarin TV, et al. Optical biopsy of human bladder neoplasia with in vivo confocal laser endomicroscopy. J Urol. 2009;182:1299–305.

35. Wu K, Liu JJ, Adams W, et al. Dynamic real-time microscopy of the urinary tract using confocal laser endomicroscopy. Urology. 2011;78:225–31.

36. Adams W, Wu K, Liu JJ, Hsiao ST, Jensen KC, Liao JC. Comparison of 2.6- and 1.4-mm imaging probes for confocal laser endomicroscopy of the urinary tract. J Endourol. 2011;25:917–21.

37. Inoue T, Murano M, Murano N, et al. Comparative study of conventional colonoscopy and pan-colonic narrow-band imaging system in the detection of neoplastic colonic polyps: a randomized, controlled trial. J Gastroenterol. 2008;43:45–50.

38. Sharma P, Bansal A, Mathur S, et al. The utility of a novel narrow band imaging endoscopy system in patients with Barrett's esophagus. Gastrointest Endosc. 2006;64:167–75.

39. Traxer O, Geavlete B, de Medina SG, Sibony M, Al-Qahtani SM. Narrow-band imaging digital flexible ureteroscopy in detection of upper urinary tract transitional-cell carcinoma: initial experience. J Endourol. 2011;25:19–23.

Diagnostic and Treatment Algorithm of Upper Tract Urothelial Carcinoma

13

Andrew I. Fishman, Lynn J. Paik, and Michael Grasso III

A.I. Fishman, MD (✉)
Department of Urology, New York Medical College,
Valhalla, NY 10595, USA
e-mail: afishman@Iupny.com

L.J. Paik, DO
Department of Urology, Lenox Hill Hospital,
New York, NY 10075, USA
e-mail: ljpaik@gmail.com

M. Grasso III
Department of Urology, New York Medical College,
Valhalla, New York, USA
e-mail: mgrasso3@earthlink.net

© Springer International Publishing Switzerland 2015
M. Grasso III, D.H. Bagley (eds.), *Upper Urinary Tract Urothelial Carcinoma*,
DOI 10.1007/978-3-319-13869-5_13

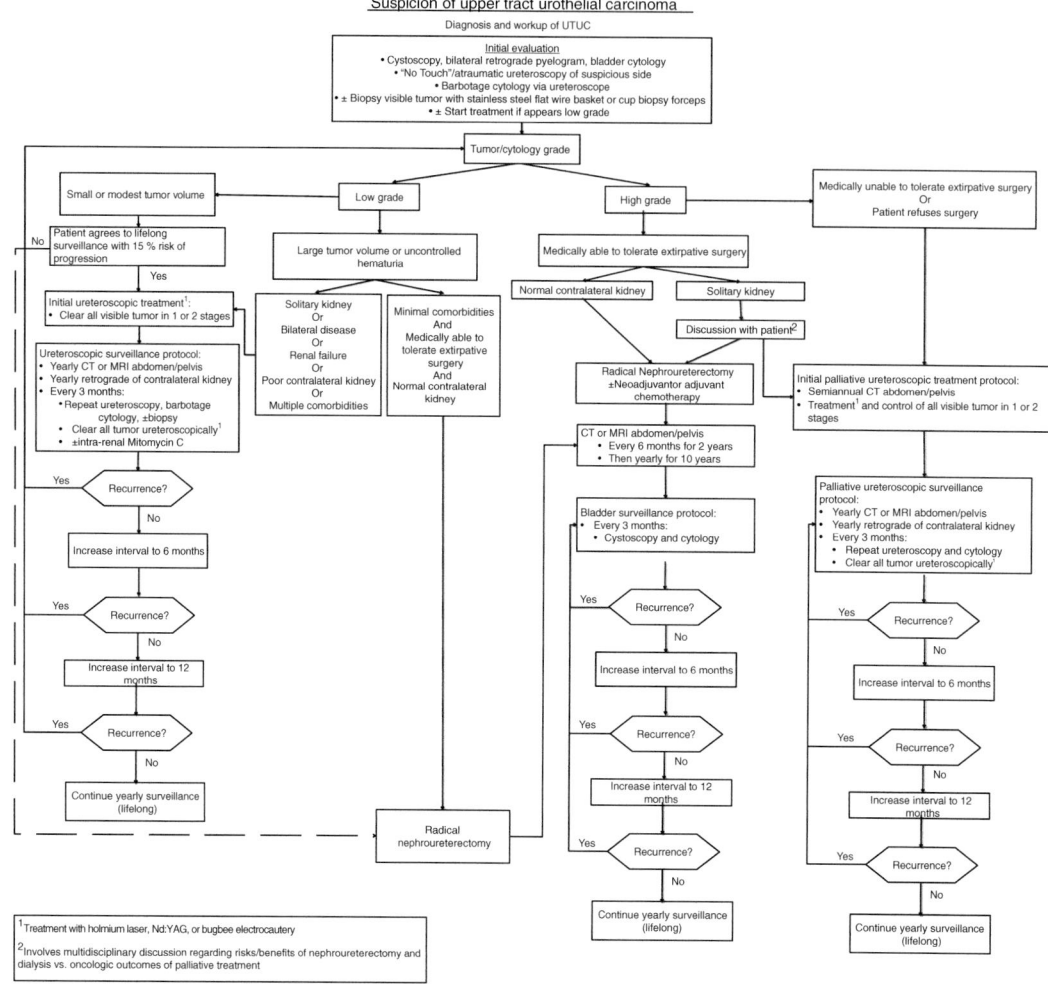

Index